Spinocerebellar Ataxia - Concepts, Particularities and Generalities

Edited by Patricia Bozzetto Ambrosi

Published in London, United Kingdom

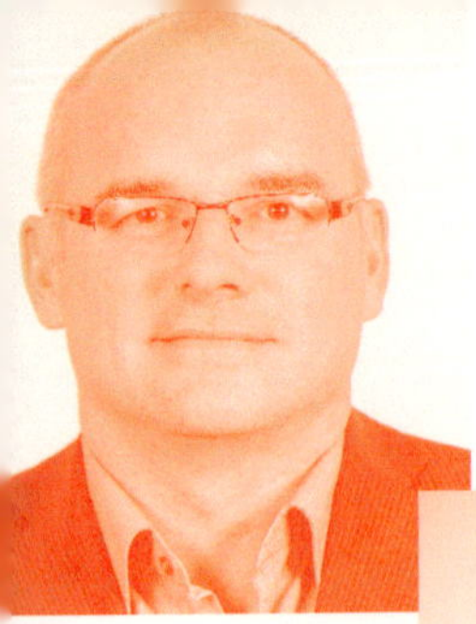
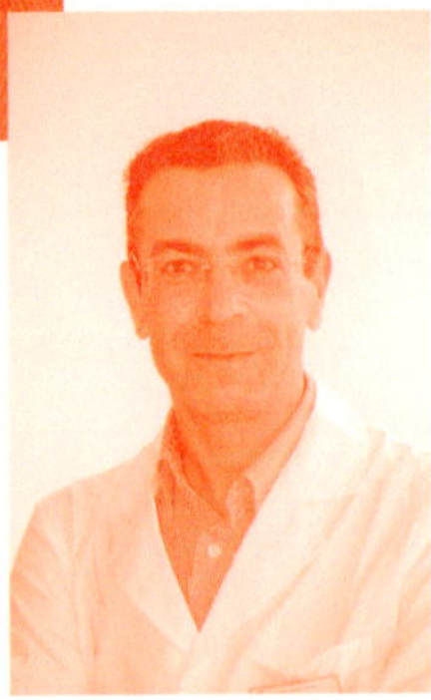
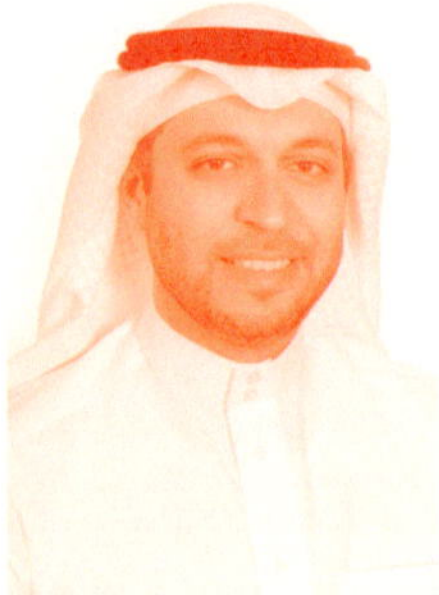
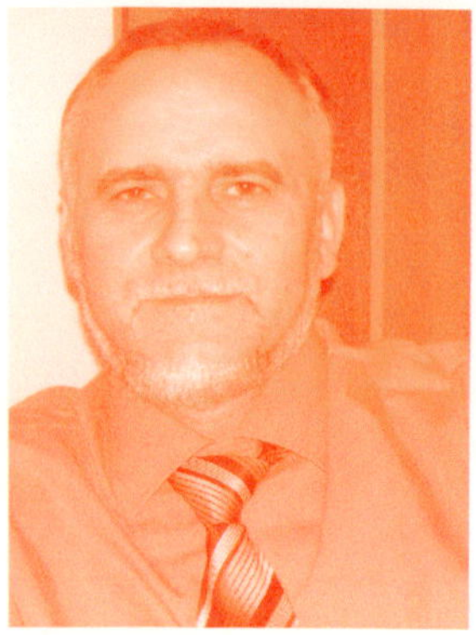
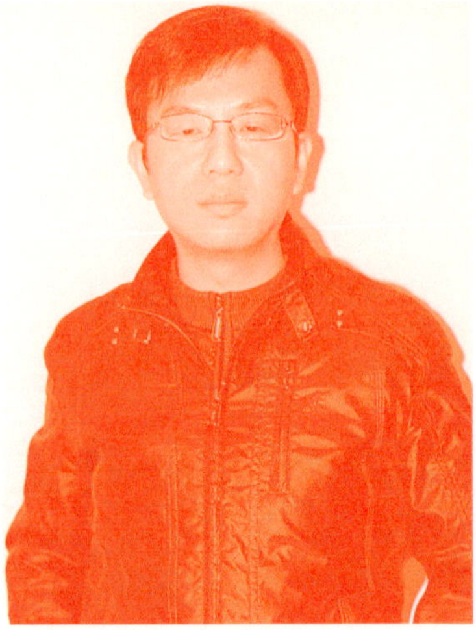
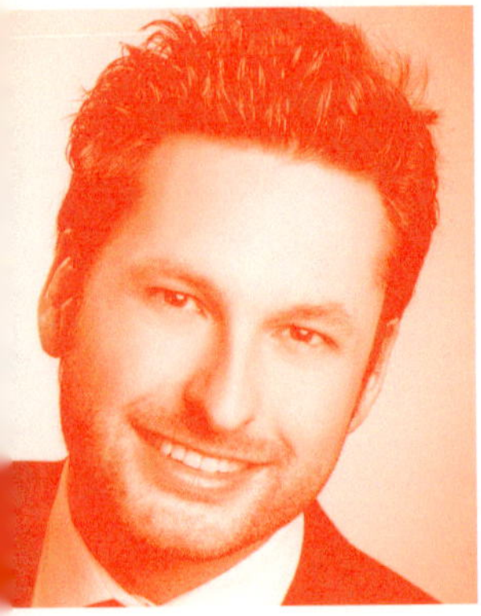
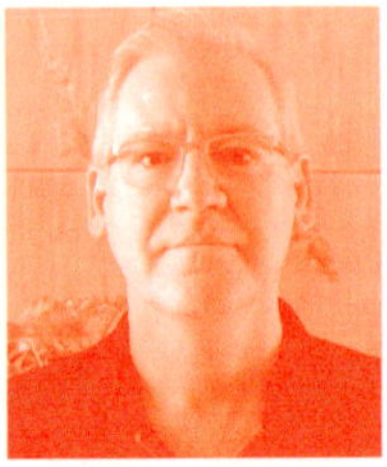

IntechOpen

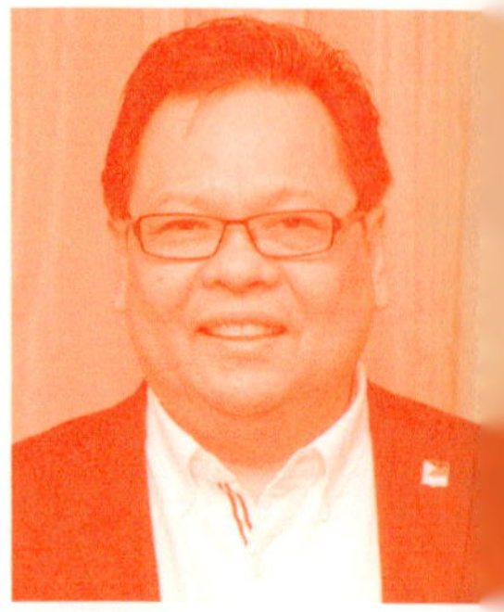
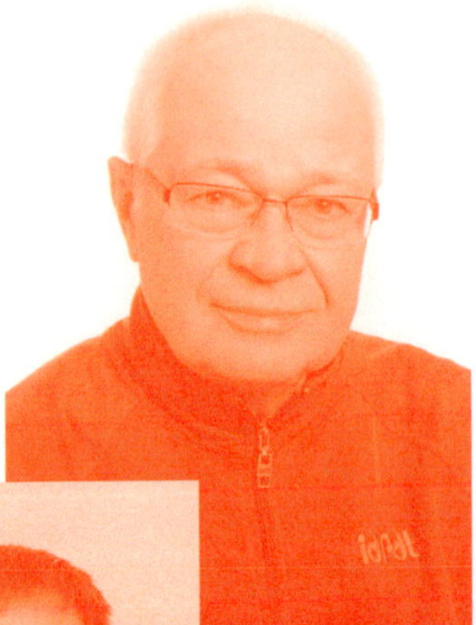
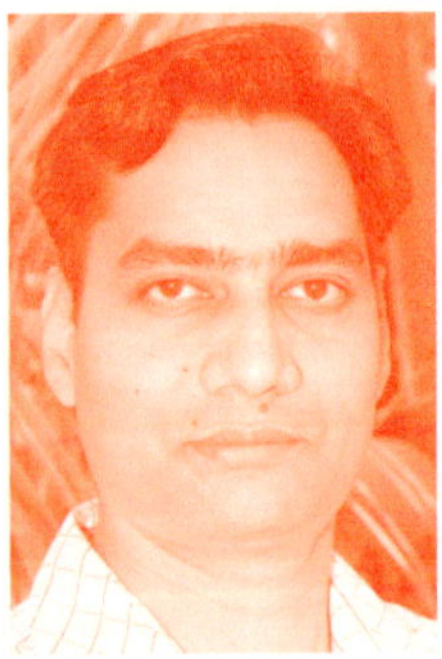
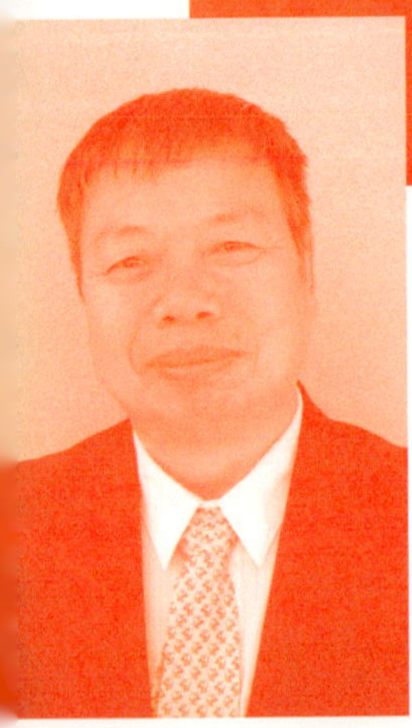
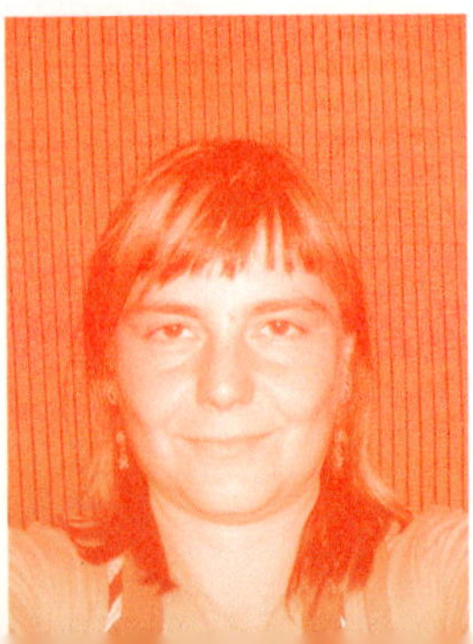
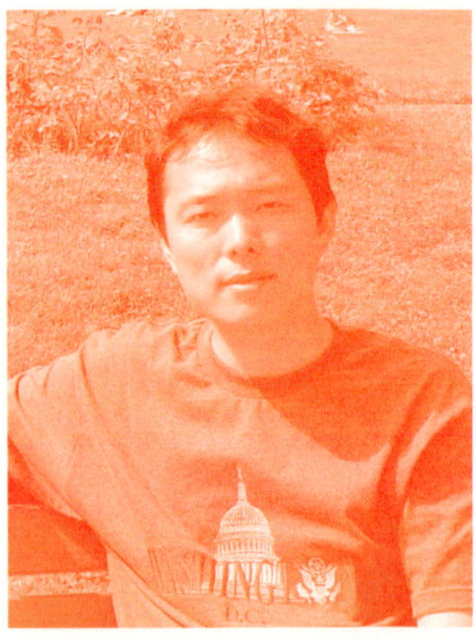

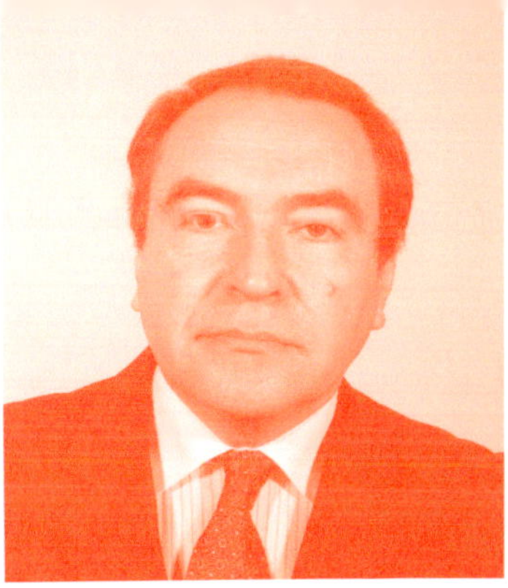
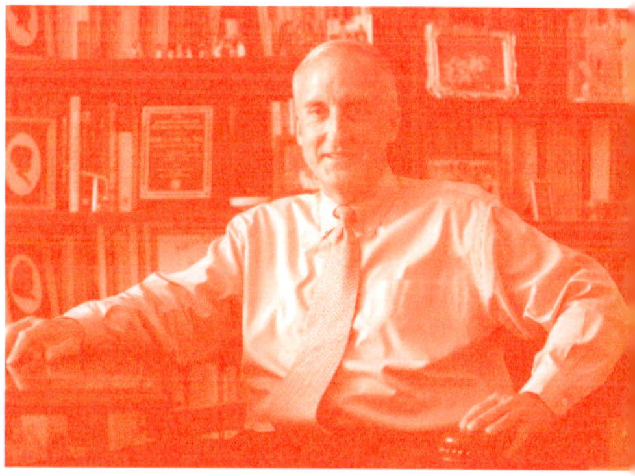
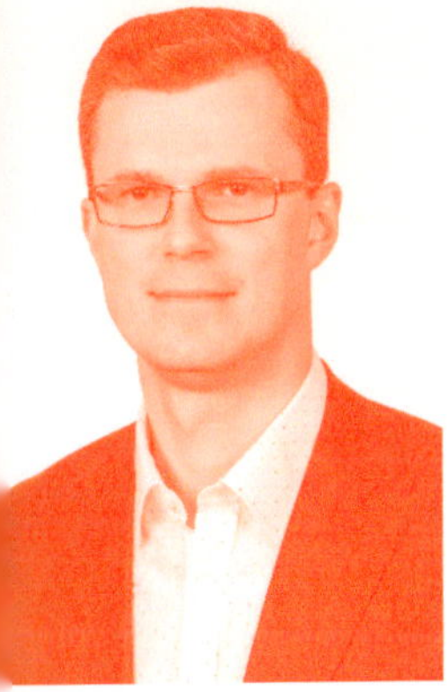
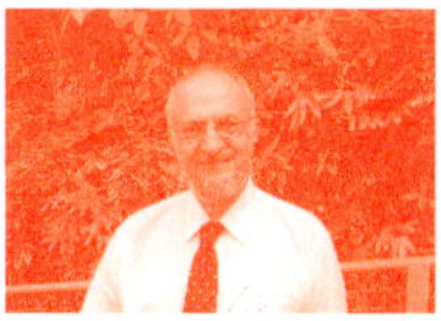
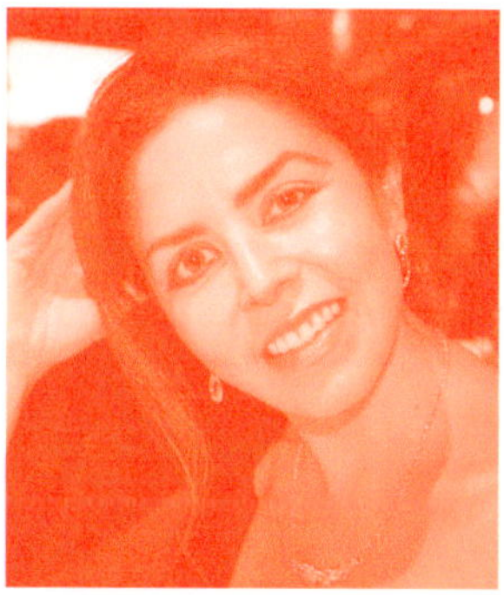

Supporting open minds since 2005

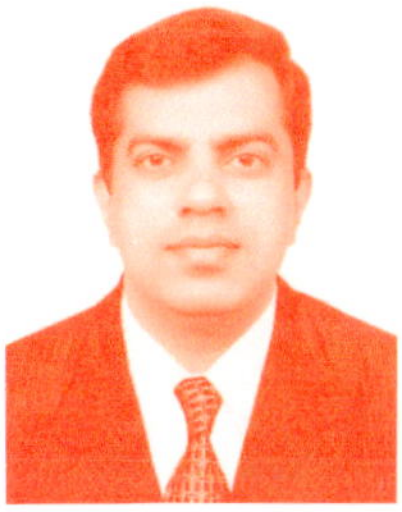
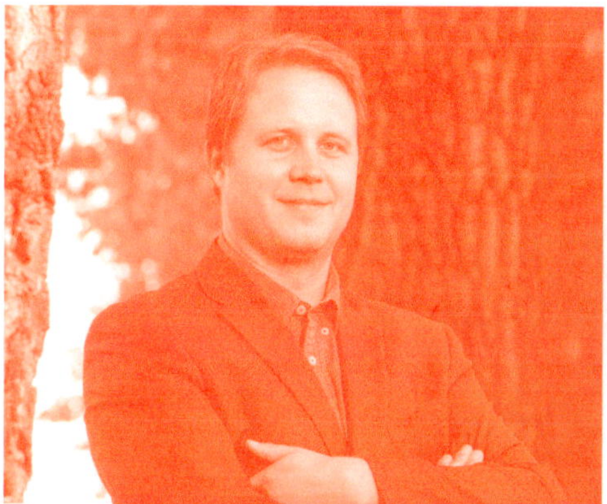
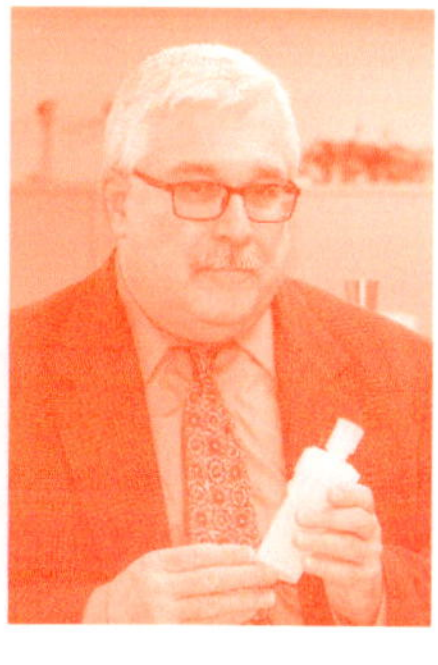
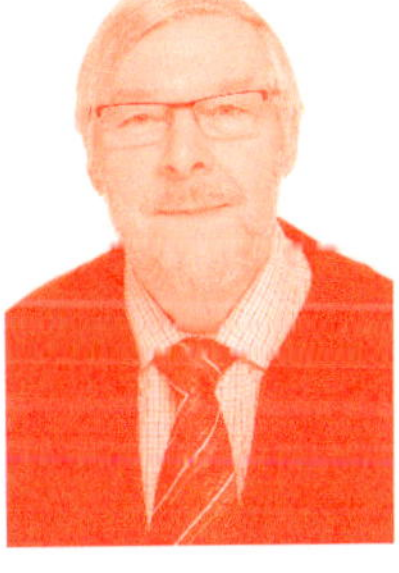
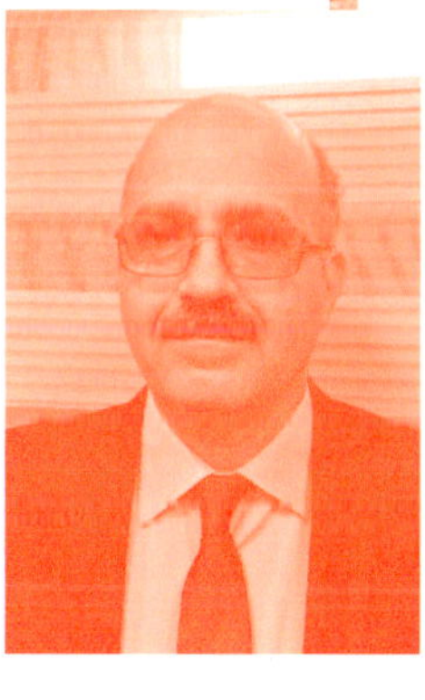
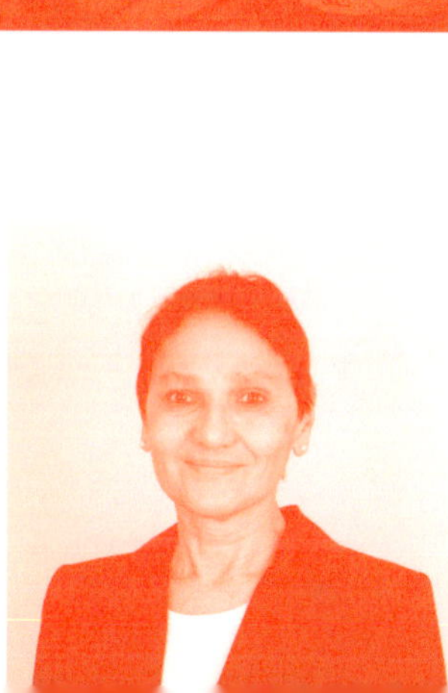
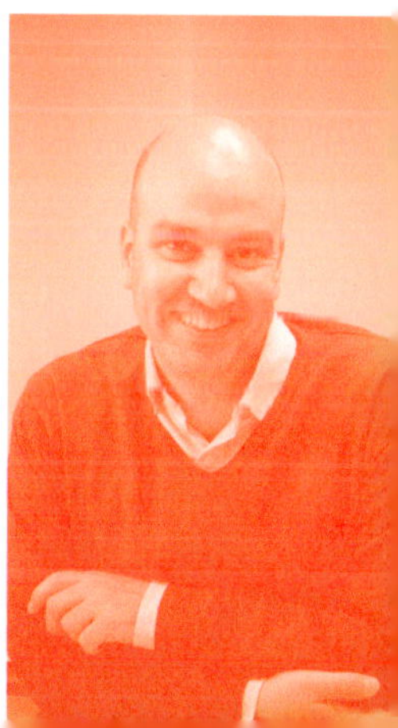

Spinocerebellar Ataxia - Concepts, Particularities and Generalities
http://dx.doi.org/10.5772/intechopen.87421
Edited by Patricia Bozzetto Ambrosi

Contributors
Kevin Triangto, Steven Setiono, Herdiman Bernard Purba, Roxana Deleanu, Rajasekhar Sajja Srinivasa Siva Naga, Akiyoshi Matsugi, Kyota Bando, Yutaka Kikuchi, Yuki Kondo, Hideki Nakano, Donnette Alicia Wright, Kadiann Peta-Gay Hewitt-Thompson, Patricia Bozzetto Ambrosi, Caroline Bozzetto Ambrosi

First published in London, United Kingdom, 2022 by IntechOpen
IntechOpen is the global imprint of INTECHOPEN LIMITED, registered in England and Wales, registration number: 11086078, 5 Princes Gate Court, London, SW7 2QJ, United Kingdom
Printed in Croatia

British Library Cataloguing-in-Publication Data
A catalogue record for this book is available from the British Library

Additional hard and PDF copies can be obtained from orders@intechopen.com

Spinocerebellar Ataxia - Concepts, Particularities and Generalities
Edited by Patricia Bozzetto Ambrosi
p. cm.
Print ISBN 978-1-83880-836-5
Online ISBN 978-1-83880-837-2
eBook (PDF) ISBN 978-1-83880-967-6

For EU product safety concerns:
IN TECH d.o.o., Prolaz Marije Krucifikse Kozulić 3, 51000 Rijeka, Croatia, info@intechopen.com or visit our website at intechopen.com.

Meet the editor

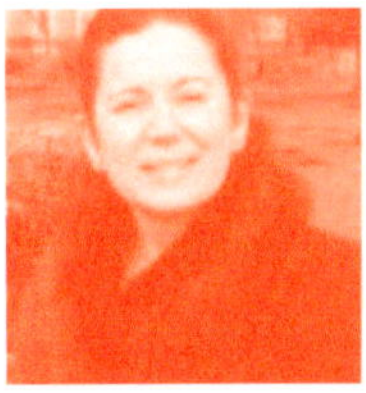

Prof. Dr. Patricia Bozzetto Ambrosi graduated with degrees in Medicine from the University of Caxias do Sul, Brazil, and the University of Rome Tor Vergata, Italy. She is a former researcher in morphophysiology at the University of Córdoba/Reina Sofia Hospital, Córdoba, Spain. She graduated in Neurology/Neurosurgery at the Hospital of Restauração, SES, Brazil, and Neuroradiology/Radiodiagnostics at Pierre and Marie Curie University, France. She holds a master's degree in Medicine from the University of Nova Lisboa, Portugal, and in Behavioral Sciences and Neuropsychiatry from the University of Pernambuco, Brazil. She also has a Ph.D. in Biological Sciences from the University of Pernambuco/Paris Diderot University, France. She is a former fellow in Interventional Neuroradiology in France at the Ophthalmological Foundation Adolphe de Rothschild, Beaujon Hospital, and Hospices Civils de Strasbourg. She was Praticien Associé in Interventional Neuroradiology at Neurologique Hospital Pierre Wertheimer, University of Lyon Claude Bernard, France, and visiting professor of the University of Paris Diderot-Neuri Beaujon. Dr. Ambrosi is an independent consultant/supervisor in neurology, neuroradiology, neuroendovascular, and imaging, and a clinical professor of medicine. She has also been an academic collaborator researcher in the Cardiovascular Department, University of Leicester, England. She has experience in innovative research for the development of new technologies and neurosciences. She is also an academic editor and reviewer of several scientific publications about neurological diseases.

Contents

Preface

Spinocerebellar ataxia (SCA) is a neurological pathology that is among the most challenging pathologies in the current medical scenario. SCA has a wide spectrum of clinical presentations, including degenerative and progressive forms with a decline in functional capacity, life-threatening characteristics, and long-standing presentation with great variability in symptoms and clinical severity. Our book addresses the background concepts, generalities, and particularities related to SCA, including clinical, neurological, genetic, and functional aspects. The book also gathers necessary information for functional classification, new approaches to medical and non-medical treatment, and rehabilitation/support, including aspects of palliative supportive care.

The book is divided into three sections. The first section, "Background: Concepts and Features" begins with Chapter 1, "Anatomy of Cerebellum." This chapter examines the functional features, main pathways, and blood supply of the cerebellum as well as clinical generalities and particularities when progressive and slow degeneration of the cerebellum occurs and certain parts of the spinal cord. Chapter 2 discusses the impact of nutrition on SCA, implementing the cyclical impact of this neurological condition on nutritional status and its corresponding impact on disease progression. It also includes recommendations and standardized guidance crucial to expanding the healthcare approach and the overall wellness of individuals with SCA.

In the second section, Chapter 3, aims to help physicians identify the activity and participation aspects of SCA, mainly around the function of mobility that can become a focus of rehabilitation intervention. Neuroplasticity through self-recognition of errors is the main physiology of recovery in SCA.

The final section deals with medical and non-medical interventions. Chapter 4 approaches the therapies of cerebellar neurons derived from human pluripotent stem cells (PSCs), from development to modeling of cerebellar ataxias. It is noteworthy that PSC technology has emerged as an important tool for the generation of different types of neurons, which are used to better understand the development and pathologies of the human nervous system. Strategies for differentiating human PSCs into cerebellar neurons are presented, followed by a perspective for their further optimization and diversification through the implementation of knowledge of cerebellar development and new cell culture approaches. The reported iPSC-derived in vitro models for cerebellar ataxias are reviewed, followed by a perspective on how to improve these models by generating and exporting cerebellar neurons. Chapter 5 presents a narrative review of rehabilitation, which is an important treatment for SCA. The lack of improvement in ataxia, motor learning deficit, and unstable balance cause incapacity for activities of daily living and restrict participation in social activities, further resulting in a disturbance in the restoration of quality of life. Finally, Chapter 6 addresses the role of palliative medicine within SCA.

Prof. Dr. Patricia Bozzetto Ambrosi
Independent Neuroradiologist and Neurologist Consultant,
Clinical Professor and Academic Researcher,
Fellow of European Academy of Neurology,
United Kingdom

Section 1

Background: Concepts and Features

Chapter 1

Anatomy of Cerebellum

Rajasekhar Sajja Srinivasa Siva Naga

Abstract

The cerebellum receives inputs from spinal cord, cerebrum, brainstem, and sensory systems of the body and controls the motor system of the body. The Cerebellum harmonizes the voluntary motor activities such as maintenance of posture and equilibrium, and coordination of voluntary muscular activity including learning of the motor behaviours. Cerebellum occupies posterior cranial fossa, and it is relatively a small part of the brain. It weighs about one tenth of the total brain. Cerebellar lesions do not cause motor or cognitive impairment. However, they cause slowing of movements, tremors, lack of equilibrium/balance. Complex motor action becomes shaky and faltering.

Keywords: Cerebellum, Spinocerebellar ataxia, Cortex, Medulla, Peduncles, Nuclei

1. Introduction

The Cerebellum is the largest part of the hindbrain and develops from the alar plates (rhombic lips) of the metencephalon.

It lies between the temporal and occipital lobes of cerebrum and the brainstem in the posterior cranial fossa. It is attached to the posterior surface of the brainstem by three large white fibre bundles. It is attached to the midbrain by superior cerebellar peduncle, pons by middle cerebellar peduncle, and medulla by inferior cerebellar peduncle.

Cerebellum is concerned with three primary functions: a) coordination of voluntary motor functions of the body initiated by the cerebral cortex at an unconscious level, b) maintenance of balance, and posture, c) Maintenance of muscle tone. It receives and integrates the sensory inputs from the cerebrum and the spinal cord necessary for a planning and smooth coordination of the movements [1].

Cerebellar lesions result in irregular and uncoordinated, awkward intentional muscle movements. Cerebellar lesions often present as occipital headache that worsen at night, nausea, vomiting and unsteadiness. On examination the patients often have bilateral papilledema, nystagmus, slight slurred speech, irregular and ataxic movements [2].

2. External features of cerebellum

Cerebellum consists three parts; two laterally located **hemispheres** joined in the midline by the **vermis** (*worm*). Somatotopy: Vermis controls the central parts of the body (trunk) and its lesions produce truncal ataxia. And each hemisphere control ipsilateral limb, and their lesion causes ataxia of ipsilateral limbs. Superior surface of the cerebellum is separated from the occipital lobe cerebrum by tentorium cerebelli of dura mater. Superior vermis protrudes above the cerebellar hemispheres whereas the inferior vermis is buried in a deep groove present between the two bulging lateral lobes. The surface of the cerebellum features highly convoluted folds(folia) that are oriented transversely. These folds are separated by fissures of variable depths. Some of the deep fissures can be used as landmarks to anatomically divide the Cerebellum into three lobes: **anterior, posterior** and **flocculonodular lobes**. On the superior surface, a deep **primary fissure** separates the small anterior lobe from the large posterior lobe. On the inferior surface, a prominent **posterolateral fissure** isolates the flocculus of cerebellar hemisphere together with the nodule of the vermis from the rest of the cerebellum as flocculonodular lobe [2].

2.1 Cerebellar lobes (Phylogenetic/Evolutionary and Functional divisions)

a. Antezrior Lobe (Spinocerebellum-Spinocerebellar tract)

- It lies anterior to the primary fissure. It regulates the muscle tone. It receives input from muscle spindles (stretch receptor) and Golgi tendon organs (GTOs) through spinocerebellar tract.

b. Posterior lobe (Neocerebellum-Corticopontocerebellar tract)

- It lies between the primary fissure and posterolateral fissure. It regulates the voluntary motor activity. It receives enormous inputs from neocortex through cortico-pontocerebellar tract.

c. Flocculonodular lobe (Vestibulocerebellum- Vestibulocerebellar tract)

- It consists of flocculus and the nodule (vermis). It regulates the maintenance of balance and posture.

2.2 Longitudinal organisation of Cerebellum

Cerebellum consists of three functional zones that are longitudinally oriented, and these zones are connected to specific cerebellar nuclei.

a. **Median (Vermal) zone** of hemisphere consists of the cortex of the vermis and it is connected to fastigial nucleus.

b. **Paramedian (Paravermal) zone** consists of the cortex of the hemisphere that is immediately adjacent to the vermis and it is connected to nucleus interpositus (Globose and Emboliform nuclei)

c. **Lateral zone** consists of cortex of the hemisphere that is exclusive of vermal and paravermal regions [3].

3. Internal structure of the cerebellum

Like the cerebral cortex, the **Cerebellum** also consists of outer shell of **grey matter** (cerebellar cortex) and the inner core **white matter**. The white matter consists of afferents and efferent fibres that go to and from the cortex. The white

DOI: http://dx.doi.org/10.5772/intechopen.97579

mater present underneath the grey mater resembles branches of a tree, hence named *arbor vitae cerebelli* (tree of life). The fibres reach the cortex in a characteristic branch like projections.

The four cerebellar nuclei are distributed deeply within the white mater in each cerebellar hemisphere. The cerebellar nuclei, while connected to the cerebellar cortex, give off the outflow form the cerebellum to the other parts of the brain. The connections are primarily to brainstem nuclei and the thalamus.

3.1 Cerebellar cortex

On the surface of the cerebellum, a highly convoluted cortex forms numerous transversely oriented folium. The cerebellar cortex is filled with cerebellar neuronal cell bodies, dendrites, and various synapses. The cortex is histologically divided into three layers:

a. Outer, **Molecular layer** (Fibre rich)

b. Middle, **Purkinje cell layer**

c. Inner, **Granule cell layer** (Granule cells)

a. **Molecular layer:** It is the outer most layer, present adjacent to the pia mater. *White fibres*: It contains dendritic arborisation of Purkinje cells and parallel fibres of Granule cells. *Cell bodies*: It contains **stellate** (outer) **cells** and **basket** (inner stellate) **cells.**

b. **Purkinjee cell layer:** It is present between the molecular and the granule cell layer. It consists of single row of cell bodies of **Purkinje cells**. The dendrites branch extensively and extend into the outer molecular layer. The dendritic branches are flattened in a single axis and are oriented at right angles to the long axis of the folium and the parallel fibres. Because of this arrangement, the branches of Purkinje fibres are perpendicularly traversed by the parallel fibres of molecular layer. The axons of Purkinje cells *form the only output* from the cerebellar cortex. Axons of the Purkinje cells end in cerebellar nuclei (dentate, emboliform, globose, fastigial) and vestibular nuclei and has an inhibitory effect (gama-aminobutyric acid, GABA) on them. Therefore, entire cerebellar output is facilitated through the inhibition of the cells of deep cerebellar nuclei.

> **Excitatory input:** Parallel fibres of granule cells (Glutamate) and climbing fibres (Aspartate) excite the Purkinje cells.
> **Inhibitory inputs:** Golgi cells, basket cells and stellate cells inhibit (GABA) the Purkinje cells.

c. **Granule cell layer:** It is present between Purkinje cell layer and the white mater of cerebellum and contains granule cells. It contains granule cells, Golgi cells, and cerebellar glomeruli. Cerebellar glomeruli are made up of granule cell dendrite, Golgi tenson axon and mossy fibre rosette. The parallel fibres of **granule cells** excite Purkinje cells, basket cells, stellate cells, Golgi cells.

> **Excitatory input:** Mossy fibres excite the granule cells.
> **Inhibitory inputs:** Golgi cells inhibit the granule cells

4. White Fibres of cerebellum

Afferents travel through cerebellar peduncles and reach the cerebellar cortical neurons to stimulate them. Based on the origin, the afferents reaching cerebellar cortex are classified as: 1) Climbing fibres, 2) Mossy fibres.

4.1 Mossy fibres

The afferent fibres (excitatory) of **spinocerebellar tract, pontocerebellar tract, and vestibulocerebellar tract** are called as mossy fibres. Mossy fibres branch and terminate in an excitatory synapse with the granule cells as mossy fibre rosette, of several folia. The axons of granule cells enter the molecular layer, through Purkinje layer and split to form two **parallel fibres** which run along the long axis of the folium. Mossy fibres excite granule cells which discharge via their parallel fibres.

Spinocerebellar tract + Olivocerebellar tract → Mossy fibres → +Granule cells → Parallel fibres

4.2 Climbing fibres

The afferent fibres (excitatory, aspartate) of **olivocerebellar tract** from contralateral inferior olivary nucleus of medulla are called as climbing fibres. They terminate on the dendrites of Purkinje cells and the deep cerebellar nuclei [4].

5. Cerebellar nuclei

Four cerebellar nuclei lie deep within the cerebellar white matter of each hemisphere. They are arranged from lateral to medial as follows:

- Dentate Nucleus (Tooth like serrated edge)
- Emboliform nucleus (Plug or Wedge-shaped)
- Globose nucleus (Spherical shaped)
- Fastigial nucleus (Peak of the Fourth ventricle: Fastigium)

5.1 Extracerebellar afferents of cerebellar nuclei

The collateral branches of Mossy fibers coming from: a) vestibular nuclei, b) reticular nuclei, c) pontine nuclei, d) spinocerebellar tract.

Among the deep cerebellar nuclei, the dentate nucleus with its crinkled bag-like appearance is the largest and the only nucleus visible to the naked eye. The dentate nucleus receives afferent fibers from the inferior olivary nucleus of the medulla, which also looks like a crinkled bag.

5.2 Intracerebellar afferents of cerebellar nuclei

Purkinje cells of the cerebellar cortex.

5.3 Efferent from Cerebellum

The majority of the efferent fibers leaving the cerebellum originate from the deep cerebellar nuclei. The efferent fibers reach: a) reticular nuclei, b) vestibular nuclei, c) red nucleus, ventral lateral nucleus of the thalamus.

6. Functional anatomy of cerebellum

Functionally, anatomically, and phylogenetically/ evolutionarily cerebellum can be divided into Archicerebellum, Paleocerebellum, Neocerebellum.

a. **Archicerebellum** consists of the flocculonodular lobe and nucleus fastigius. It is evolutionarily the first one to develop. **Connections:** Vestibulocerebellar: vestibular receptors of labyrinths, vestibular, and reticular nuclei through inferior cerebellar peduncle, spinal cord. **Function:** Maintenance of balance (equilibrium), posture, and coordination of eye movements.

Bilateral balance control by Archicerebellum

Superior colliculus + Striate cortex ➔Inferior cerebellar peduncle➔ Flocculonodular lobe➔Purkinje fibres (cerebellar cortex)➔Fastigeal Nucleus➔ Inferior cerebellar peduncle➔ IPSILATERAL & CONTRALATERAL vestibular nuclei + Reticular formation ➔ Vestibulospinal tract, Reticulospinal tracts➔ Spinal cord.

b. **Paleocerebellum** consists of the vermis, paravermis, fastigial nucleus, emboliform nucleus. **Function:** Controls the tone and posture of the trunk and proximal limb muscles through the vermal-cerebellar pathway. **Connections: Spinocerebellar:** Spinal cord and red nucleus through inferior and superior cerebellar peduncle.

Contralateral muscle tone and posture control by Paleocerebellum

Receptors of Muscle, Joint, Skin➔ Dorsal Spinocerebellar tract ➔ Inferior cerebellar peduncle➔IPSILATERAL vermis +paravermis➔ Globose nucleus + emboliform Nucleus+ Fastigial nucleus➔ Superior cerebellar peduncle➔ CONTRALATERAL red Nucleus➔ Rubrospinal tract.

Receptors of Muscle, Joint, Skin ➔ Ventral spinocerebellar tract➔ Superior cerebellar peduncle➔ IPSILATERL vermis+ paravermis➔ Globose nucleus+ Emboliform nucleus➔ Superior cerebellar peduncle➔ CONTRALATERAL Red nucleus➔ Rubrospinal tract.

c. **Neocerebellum** consists of the remaining cerebellar hemisphere (except pyramid and uvula) and dentate nucleus. **Function:** Controls the highly skilled muscle coordination and trajectory, speed, and force of movements. **Connections: Cortico-pontocerebellar:** Pontine nuclei, cerebral cortex.

Coordination of movement by Neocortex

Planning+ execution of movement➔Cerebral cortex➔ corticopontine fibres➔ Pontine nuclei➔ Pontocerebellar fibres➔ CONTRALATERAL middle cerebellar peduncle➔ Lateral parts of cerebellar hemi spheres ➔ Dentate nucleus➔ Superior cerebellar peduncle➔ Contralateral Red nucleus (rubrothalamic cells) + Ventral lateral nucleus of Thalamus➔ motor cortex of frontal lobe of cerebrum➔ Corticospinal tract+ Corticobulbar tract

7. Cerebellar Peduncles

These are the white fibre bundles that join the different parts of the brain stem with the cerebellum.

7.1 Superior cerebellar peduncle (Midbrain➔ Cerebellum)

Afferent fibers from:

- *Spinal cord* (**Ventral spinocerebellar tract**, **Major input**)
- *Tectum of the midbrain* (Tectocerebellar fibers)
- *Hypothalamus* (Hypothalamocerebellar fibers)
- *Locus ceruleus* (Ceruleocerebellar fibers)

Efferent fibers to:

- Globose and emboliform nuclei➔ contralateral *red nucleus* (Cerebellorubral fibers)
- Dentate nucleus➔ contralateral *red nucleus* (Dentatorubral fibers)
- Dentate nucleus ➔ contralateral *Thalamus*: Ventral lateral nucleus (**Dentatothalamic fibers, Major output**)
- Dentate nucleus➔ contralateral *inferior olivary nucleus* (Cerebello-olivary fibres)
- Nucleus fastigius ➔ *Reticular nuclei* (Cerebelloreticular fibers)

7.2 Middle cerebellar peduncle (Pons ➔ Cerebellum)

Afferent fibers from:

- Contralateral *pontine nuclei* (**Cortico-ponto-cerebellar fibers, Major input**)
- *Ipsilateral Reticular formation*➔ vermis (Reticulocerebellar fibers)
- *Raphe nuclei of pons* (Seratogenic fibers)

Efferent fibers to: No efferents.

7.3 Inferior cerebellar peduncle

Afferent fibers from:

- Ipsilateral *thoracic nucleus of Spinal cord*, Clarke's column (**Dorsal spinocerebellar tract, Major input**).
- Ipsilateral *accessory cuneate nucleus* (**Cuneocerebellar tract, Major input**),
- *Inferior olivary nucleus* (**Olivocerebellar tract**➔ climbing fibers, **Major input**)
- Contralateral *medial and dorsal accessory olivary nucleus* (Parolivocerebellar tract),

- *Vestibular nuclei* (Vestibulocerebellar tract)
- *Lateral and paramedian reticular nuclei* (Reticulocerebellar tract)

Efferent fibers to:

- Ipsilateral flocculonodular lobe ➔ bilateral *Vestibular nuclei* (Cerebellovestibular fibers)
- Bilateral Fastigial nuclei➔ *reticular formation* of pons and medulla (Cerebelloreticluar fibers)
- *Inferior olivary nucleus* (Cerebello-olivary fibers)

7.4 Major pathways

Cerebellum-Cerebrum-Cerebellum circuit
Purkinje cells ➔ Dentate nucleus ➔ superior cerebellar peduncle➔ dentatothalamic tract➔ Contralateral ventral lateral nucleus of Thalamus ➔ primary motor cortex of precentral gyrus (Brodmann's area 4, motor strip)➔ corticopontine tract➔ pontine nuclei➔ pontocerebellar tract➔ contralateral cerebellar cortex➔ mossy fibers.

8. Blood supply of Cerebellum

The cerebellum is supplied by posterior circulation originated from vertebral arteries. The vertebral artery gives rise to the posterior inferior cerebellar artery (PICA), which supplies the posterior part of the inferior surface of the cerebellum. The basilar artery gives rise to the anterior inferior cerebellar artery (AICA), which supplies the anterior part of the inferior surface. The superior cerebellar artery (SCA) supplies the superior surface of the cerebellum [1].

9. In the clinic

9.1 Cerebellar disorders

a. Hypotonia (reduced muscle tone) and ataxia (loss of coordinated muscular movements) (Most characteristic signs)

b. Dysequilibrium: loss of balance, gait, and trunk ataxia

c. Dyssynergia (loss of coordinated muscle activity): a) Dysmetria (inability to do the finger-nose test), b) Intentional tremor on voluntary movements, c) Dysdiadochokinesia (inability to do rapid alternating repetitive movements).

d. Ipsilateral reduced tendon reflexes

e. Asthenia

f. Cerebellar Nystagmus (coarse)

9.2 Midline lesions

The midline lesions of the cerebellum (vermis) cause loss of control of trunk posture resulting in truncal ataxia. Patients present with the inability to sit or stand, as there would be involuntary swinging of the body back and forth to stabilize around the center of gravity.

9.3 Unilateral cerebellar lesions

Cerebellar tracts **do not decussate** like the cerebrum. The symptoms (limb ataxia) produced by the lesions of cerebellar hemispheres are ipsilateral. Unilateral lesions of cerebellar hemispheres cause ipsilateral loss of arm or leg coordination resulting in an unsteady gait (No motor or sensory loss). Limb ataxia can be tested by asking the patient to do a "**heel to shin**" test. When patients with limb ataxia try to walk, the body has difficulty coordinating muscle movements, leading to shifting **the center of gravity**. When there is a fall due to a significant shift in the center of gravity, the fall is usually towards the same **side of the lesion**. The patient often compensates for this by lowering their center of gravity by **wide stepped gait** [5].

9.4 Bilateral cerebellar dysfunction

Bilateral cerebellar dysfunction causes the following symptoms:

a. **Dysarthria**: slurring of speech

b. **Cerebellar ataxia**: unsteady, wide-based, staggering gait and incoordination of both arms

c. **Nystagmus**: involuntary rhythmic to-and-fro movements of the eyeball. Symptoms increase when the gaze is pointed to the side of the lesion.

Diseases in which cerebellum is affected bilaterally: a) hypothyroidism, b) alcoholic intoxication, c) multiple sclerosis, d) degenerative diseases, e) metabolic disorders).

Charcot's triad: A characteristic combination of nystagmus, dysarthria, and intentional tremor are observed in multiple sclerosis.

9.5 Other causes of cerebellar dysfunction

Tumours (Astrocytoma, Medulloblastoma, Ependymomas), Hypertensive hemorrhage, cerebellar infarctions.

9.6 Cerebellar dysfunction + Hydrocephalus

Cerebellar infarctions (edema), cerebellar tumors compressing IVth ventricle.

9.7 Points to ponder

Anterior vermis syndrome, Posterior vermis syndrome, Hemispheric syndrome [5].

10. Conclusion

Cerebellum consists of median vermis and prominent lateral hemispheres. It forms the roof of the fourth ventricle behind the brain stem. It is attached to the parts of brainstem by cerebellar peduncles which are large white fibre bundles carrying afferent and efferent fibres of cerebellum. Afferent systems of cerebellum include climbing fibres and mossy fibres. It also receives fibres from brainstem reticular formation. Climbing fibres are connected to the contralateral inferior olivary nucleus of medulla oblongata, at one end, and the proximal dendrites of a single Purkinjee cell in the cerebellar cortex, at the other end. Mossy fibres are connected to spinal cord, brain stem, at one end and multiple Purkinjee cells of cerebellar cortex at another end.

11. Cerebellum and Spinocerebellar ataxia

Case study: 55 old male presents with a history of poor hand coordination, slurred speech, rapid eye movements, reduced intellectual function. Physical examination reveals cerebellar ataxia, spasticity, negative Babinski sign. Brain CT scan showed mild cerebral and marked cerebellar atrophy.

Diagnosis: Spinocerebellar ataxia.

12. Spinocerebellar ataxia

Introduction: Spinocerebellar ataxias (SCA), are a group of hereditary ataxias transmitted by autosomal dominant inheritance, in which there is a progressive and slow degeneration of cerebellum and certain parts of spinal cord. Among the many types of SCAs, they are classified based on the gene mutation responsible for a specific type of SCA. The types are described as SCA1 through SCA40.

Symptoms: The signs and symptoms across the different types generally include abnormal speech (dysarthria), uncoordinated walk (gait), poor hand-eye coordination, vision problems and difficulty in processing, learning and remembering information. The main symptom include ataxia, where smooth coordination of voluntary motor functions is lost, and there is also nystagmus where the vestibulo-cerebellar fibres and vestibulo-cerebellum are involved. Owing to the degenerative nature of the disease, not only dorsal and ventral spinocerebellar fibres carrying proprioceptive fibres from skeletal muscles and joints, almost all the functions of the cerebellum are affected in Spinocerebellar ataxias.

Etiology: Certain types of SCA are caused due to mutation called trinucleotide repeat expansion, where a particular segment of DNA is repeated number of times beyond the tolerable limit. Such nucleotide repeats are unstable and alter their length while passing through generations and often lead to early age onset of the disease. The risk of transmission of the disease from the affected generation to the next is 50%.

Diagnosis: If the disease-causing mutation is known then the carrier testing for at-risk relatives and prenatal testing can be done to diagnose the disease.

Treatment: There is no specific treatment for SCA. For ataxia, physiotherapy to strengthen the muscles can be done. Physical aids such as crutches and walkers can be used to assist daily activity of the patient [2].

Author details

Rajasekhar Sajja Srinivasa Siva Naga
Department of Anatomy, Jawaharlal Institute of Postgraduate Medical Education and Research, Puducherry, India

*Address all correspondence to: drsrinivas83@gmail.com

References

[1] Gray's Anatomy. 41st edition. London: Elsevier; 2016:331-348.

[2] Grays Clinical Neuroanatomy. Philadelphia: Elsevier; 2011: 229-244

[3] Snells Clinical Neuroanatomy. Philadelphia: Wolters Kluwer;2019:229-48.

[4] Fitzgerald's Clinical Neuroanatomy and Neuroscience. 7th Edition. New York: Elsevier;2016: 38-39.

[5] Klockgether T, Mariotti C, Paulson HL. Spinocerebellar ataxia. Nat Rev Dis Primers. 2019;5:24. https://doi.org/10.1038/s41572-019-0074-3

Chapter 2

Impact of Nutrition in Spinocerebellar Ataxia

Donnette Alicia Wright and
Kadiann Peta-Gay Hewitt-Thompson

Abstract

This chapter explores the link between the health outcomes of spinocerebellar ataxia and diet and nutrition as well as overall quality of life and well-being that is achieved as a result of nutritional support and nutritional profile. Spinocerebellar ataxia is a hereditary condition characterized by degenerative changes to parts of the brain, extending to the spinal cord, that affects mobility and voluntary actions. Due to the deteriorating impact of this neurological disorder, the management of health and wellness of the individual is imperative in stemming physiological decline and morbidity. The connections between dietary intake, quality of life and well-being are important components of the health response in providing optimum health outcomes for clients diagnosed with spinocerebellar ataxia. Consequently, an examination of factors that impede, promote and generally affect dietary intake, nutritional status and profile is essential towards improving disease related quality of life and morbidity and mortality risk. The cyclical impact of the neurological condition on nutritional status and its corresponding impact on disease progression is an important exploratory point. Finally, recommendations and standardized guidance are crucial to expanding the health care approach and the overall wellness of individuals with spinocerebellar ataxia.

Keywords: nutritional support, quality of life, muscle strength, dysphagia, weight control and wellness

1. Introduction

1.1 Methodology and literature review

A content analysis of the literature, especially produced over the last decade, was carried out exploring the condition spinocerebellar ataxia and the possible impact that diet and nutrition may have on the outcome of the condition, utilizing the keywords as a guide. The paper was presented in sections concerning diet and wellness, analyzing each concept and the relationship between diet, nutrition, and spinocerebellar ataxia especially in light of quality of life and wellness.

2. Overview of spinocerebellar ataxia and diet and nutrition

Spinocerebellar Ataxia is a heterogeneous group of neurodegenerative ataxic disorders with autosomal dominant inheritance. It is an inherited progressive disorder with clinical features including loss of balance and coordination accompanied by slurred speech. The clinical outcome of this disease is usually manifested in adulthood [1, 2]. This condition is similar to many non-communicable diseases insomuch as it is not transmissible from personal contact and has significant impact on quality of life and wellness. Considering the deteriorating neurological features of the condition, health and wellness maintenance is paramount. Diet and nutrition is featured heavily in its effect on clinical outcomes of this condition. Spinocerebellar Ataxia may have important health impact and nutritional risk profile effect due challenges with swallowing, dysphagia, dependence in meal preparations, muscle and coordination challenges. These physiological changes that are characteristic of spinocerebellar ataxia impact dietary intake and negatively affect lean body mass [3, 4]. Importantly weight loss is a predictor of morbidity risk where sepsis and concomitant illnesses were measured outcome criteria [5]. As a consequence of these physical changes and nutritional impact, the healthcare team must be responsive to the special needs of this cohort of individuals to stem possible negative outcomes. A focus on diet and wellness may accrue to significant health benefits in this population.

Diet and wellbeing are pervasive concepts impacting sociology, psychology, medicine, and human thought. Their relationship to health and happiness are significant to human development and livelihood. This chapter explores the connection between diet and wellbeing especially as they contribute to or impact health generally and particularly that of clients diagnosed with spinocerebellar ataxia. There are important factors that create the link between diet and wellness and include dietary intake, quality of life and wellbeing. The bridge between these concepts will contribute to a better understanding of the impact of diet and wellness and provide summative recommendations for the maintenance of health especially in individuals with neurological disorders such as spinocerebellar ataxia.

2.1 Dietary intake

Dietary intake is the food and nutrient consumed by an individual daily to maintain life, health, and functionality. Dietary intake is guided by set of recommendations/standards for the daily intake of nutrients and other food components based on the recommended daily allowances. These measurements are used to assess or track food, nutrient or any non-nutritional intake by individuals. The main purpose for assessing an individual's dietary intake is for nutritional screening and surveillance, which can be used to guide research. In individuals with neurological disorders, resting energy expenditure due to hypermetabolism is increased [6]. Resting energy expenditure is the caloric requirement of an individual needed to maintain life and the function of essential organs and systems at rest. It is an important feature of health management in people with neurological illness. Moreover, it is imperative that caregivers and the health care team manage caloric needs in this population, since under supply of energy increases health risks in this vulnerable group of individuals.

2.2 Quality of life

The World Health Organization defines "Quality of Life as an individual's perception of their position in life in the context of the culture and value systems in which they live and in relation to their goals, expectations, standards and concerns" [7]. The quality of life can be affected by an individual's physical health, psychological state, their personal beliefs and social relationships in relation to significant features of their environment. The Centers for Disease Control and Prevention views quality of life as a concept that can be applied to various disciplines to evaluate important aspects of individuals' lives. The concept is usually defined differently for each discipline. The concept of health-related quality of life has been explored since the 1900s. It evaluates a person's perception of their physical and mental health in relation to their health status and risks, social support and their socioeconomic status. Health- related quality of life also includes the community by identifying the resources, practices and policies of the community that may have an influence on the population's health perceptions and how well they function [8]. Importantly, in spinocerebellar ataxia many variables help to determine quality of life such as the capacity to carry out activities of living, the level of pain or discomfort and the independence to manage self care, Furthermore, the evidence considers disease related quality of life as an important element in neurological disorders and spinocerebellar ataxia in particular. This element of quality of life examines the progression of the disease relative the activities and competencies that the client retains [9]. The greater the physical independence, self care independence, the fewer the neurological deficit along with higher levels of comfort the higher the levels of general quality of life and disease related quality of life [9]. Nutrition and diet are inextricable to quality of life in these patients, so much as well balanced diets, lower health risks, meets energy needs and is associated with reductions in the progression of the disease. These concepts are explored in greater detail in the remainder of the chapter.

2.3 Wellbeing

The concept of well-being is usually viewed in a positive way for individuals as it indicates that they perceive that their lives are functioning well. An individual that has good living conditions such as proper housing and are employed is essential to their well-being [8]. Well-being is also recognized state where an individual experiences good health, happiness and prosperity, which includes their good mental health, having the ability to manage stress, satisfaction with their lives and the feeling that they have a meaning and purpose in life. Most people aim to achieve well-being because it represents positivity and general health [10].

The quality of life and wellness of an individual with a neurological disorder are affected by a cyclical relationship between nutrition and the disease state. Where poor nutrition is thought to exacerbate the clinical features of the disease and worsened diseases states negatively impact on nutritional risk profile. Specifically, chewing and swallowing difficulties affecting nutrient intake where suboptimal calorie intake is achieved. Furthermore, biochemical and physiology factors of neurological diseases in general and spinocerebellar ataxia in particular affect nutritional status through limited nutrient absorption and utilization, and physiological process affecting gross dietary intake including infection, depression, muscle atrophy, rigidity, tremor, dyskinesia, reluctance to feed, and dysphagia [6]. The combination of these factors may lead to undesired weight loss with worsened risk of infection, and sepsis. Furthermore, poorer nutritional states are associated with worsened ataxia, dyskinesia and tremors. Therefore, it is imperative to evaluate nutritional intake and specifically, caloric intake and expenditure of individuals properly in order to improve the quality of life and enhance health outcomes in clients with neurological diseases.

2.4 Factors that affect dietary intake

There are many factors that can have a positive or negative impact on an individual's dietary intake. The amount and quality of dietary intake is directly linked to nutritional profile of individuals. Considering the need for appropriate quantities of micronutrients and macronutrients to support nutritional wellbeing, the factors underpinning nutritional intake is essential for review. Some of the most significant factors that impact dietary intake are appetite, importation, physical condition, built environment and health conditions. These factors will be explored in detail with a view to understanding how positive health outcomes can be accrued. Furthermore, these factors will be examined more closely in the context of neurological diseases and spinocerebellar ataxia.

The factors impacting dietary intake are expansive and are summarized in **Figure 1**.

In many countries, especially developing countries, meals are heavily dependent on importation. However, during a pandemic importation is unreliable and unstable. As a result, these countries are at a higher risk of food shortage [12], which will impact national dietary intake. This means that there may be acute or chronic impact on individual access to food primarily resulting in reduced dietary intake. A pandemic also impacts wages, whether through job loss, reduced working hours. The household purchasing power may be diminished creating impaired food access and decreased dietary intake based on the financial challenges brought on by the pandemic [12]. While importation is not controlled at the individual level, it has important personal impact. Spinocerebellar ataxia has been significantly associated with weight loss and BMI decline due to increases in metabolic demand. The risk of weight loss worsens with disease progression [13]. Importantly, weight loss and BMI decline are treated with regularly adequate intake of energy at the estimated levels to meet total daily energy expenditure. This means that efforts must be made by health care workers, families and government to facilitate safe, and adequate access to food so that energy supply may be appropriate in this population. Importation therefore has a tangential impact on the quality of life of individuals with spinocerebellar ataxia. This exists where importation affects food access, access affects dietary intake, which affects energy balance and body weight. If weight is suboptimal, individuals with ataxia are at greater health risk and the reverse is true when weight is ideal.

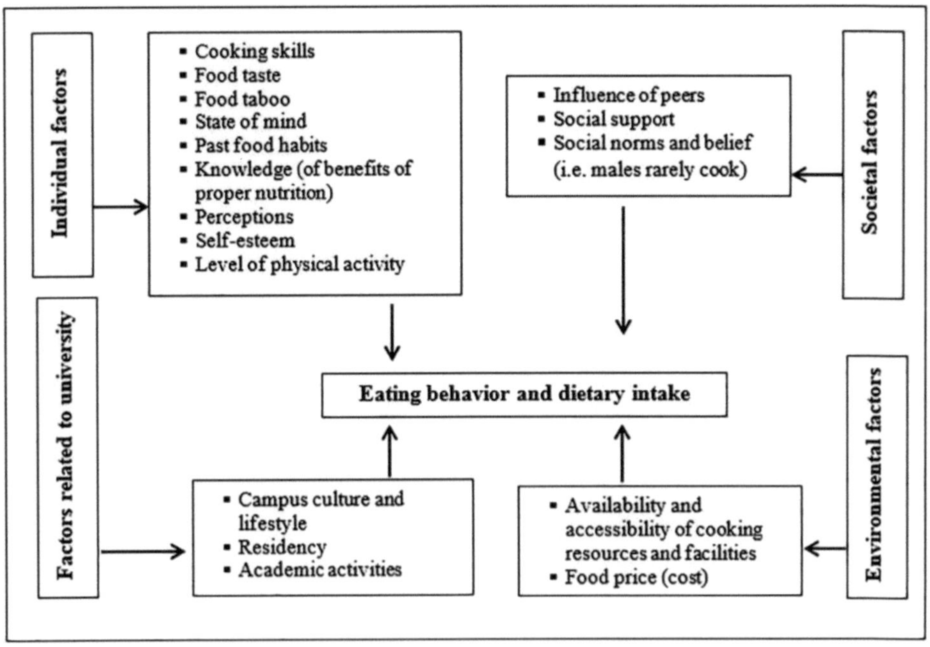

Figure 1.
Factors affecting dietary intake [11], p. 6.

There are some health conditions that affect an individual's dietary intake; that may range from challenges with digestion and absorption of nutrients or side effects from prescribed medications that interfere with absorption and utilization of nutrients and dietary adjustments may be needed in medical nutrition therapy for specified health conditions. As part of the treatment of some conditions, clients may be required to eat smaller portions, restrict some food or nutrients, or limit the amount they can tolerate. Clients with spinocerebellar ataxia are similarly afflicted. The condition is reported to impact swallowing capacity, digestion, and nutrient storage, especially fat ([6]; Ko, Qu, Black, & Tso, 2020). Some micronutrients including niacin, thiamine and tocopherol have high risk of deficiency in clients with spinocerebellar ataxia [14–16]. Consequently, nutritional support at times can be adjusted and specially formulated to meet their needs. In some instances where digestion is limited, elemental dietary formulations, texture modifications to support swallowing difficulties may be offered, or where gastrointestinal intake is severely restricted parenteral nutritional application may be necessary.

Nutrition and dietary intake have been established as major factors influencing the quality of life of patients diagnosed with spinocerebellar ataxia. Consequently, it is important to expand the dialog of nutrition in understanding how wellness is affected through dietary influence in this unique population. A major element of physical wellbeing is nutritional status which is directly proportional to the quality of dietary intake. Moreover, social, and emotional wellbeing are affected by dietary intake and nutritional status directly due to the components of food and indirectly because of the perceptions associated with the evaluation of personal nutritional status. Several factors affect dietary intake and include but are not limited to appetite, physiological development, health condition, the built environment, effects of a pandemic and social family settings. These factors will be explored in detail.

2.5 Appetite

Appetite is an individual's desire to eat food, the body's biological response to a lack of food is hunger. However, an individual's appetite can rise and fall due to various factors, sometimes causing people to eat less or more than their body needs [17]. Appetite can be affected by one's diet, mental health, pregnancy, medications or other health conditions. An individual experiencing a decrease in appetite may lead to a concordant decrease in the general desire to eat food and thus the person may consume less food and nutrients. Appetite is also an important factor impacting the nutritional status of patients with spinocerebellar ataxia. Appetite is primarily affected by the pharmacotherapy approaches used to manage/treat the condition. Drugs including Varenicline and Riluzole are used in the treatment of the neurological features of dystonia and ataxia [18]. The medications are reported to negatively impact on appetite and may potentiate weight loss. These concerns are necessary to be addressed systemically in view of the risks associated with weight loss in spinocerebellar ataxia. Corrective actions including eating by the clock, small frequent meals, colorful and attractive meals, and appetite stimulants may be important to address these appetite changes.

In the general population several personal and psychological factors were examined as factors that contributed to caloric intake. Hunger, appetite, and satiety were identified as important contributors to dietary intake among this population. Appetite was thought to relate to the psychological drive to eat [19]. There remains a concern regarding the factors that regulate appetite but dietary factors including protein and caloric load have been identified as features that influence satiety. At the alternate end of the spectrum, poor appetite is reported as a factor that affects the quality and quantity of food intake in older adults and influences health outcome and morbidity risk [20]. Markedly appetite exerts an important influence across the lifespan and influences nutritional status and wellness. Appetite may also be affected by the capacity to coordinate movements and feed self especially among the psychological influences. In spinocerebellar ataxia, physiological outcomes including uncoordinated actions limit feeding independence may contribute to reductions in appetite [6, 18, 21]. As medications are introduced to correct physiological impact in these neurological conditions caution needs to be exercised in view of the physical impact that pharmacotherapy may have on appetite. Ultimately, a tight balance must be reached between the management of physical limitations to feeding and the impact on appetite, and pharmacological approaches to managing coordination and their impact on appetite. This must be done with careful observations of diet and appetite especially as the impact on weight balance and health related quality of life.

2.6 The built environment

Social changes that have led to structural advances have improved the quality of life of the global population. These changes had led to positive financial impact, changes in commerce, trading, and travel. Conversely, it has had instrumental impact on diet and nutritional intake. Furthermore, even the dynamic of the rural population has changed. Several scholars are identifying that caution should be introduced when these benefits are examined. As the referenced changes have also been recognized as significant drivers of changes in dietary quality, where wealth has led to increased dietary intake, particularly energy and serving sizes [22]. Urbanization has led to reduction in the value of home gardens, reduction in the reliance on agrarian subsistence with resulting declines in the consumption of complex carbohydrates [23]. There is also a notable increased in energy dense, nutrient poor and processed foods. Importantly as well, statisticians have associated the structural changes with dietary changes and with significant steep increases in non-communicable diseases, and sharp declines in quality of life. Moreover, there is a concern with changes in the built environment and green spaces for exercise and physical activity. With automation and innovations in construction, there has been a corresponding decline in physical activity with an increased risk of non-communicable diseases [24]. Physical activity is directly related to nutritional status as physical activity helps to create a balance between caloric intake and expenditure especially as weight maintenance in adulthood is desired. In clients with spinocerebellar ataxia muscle strength, disuse, and incoordination impact on the capacity to engage in the physical activity [6]. Notably, physical activity has been linked to improvement in the quality of life of patients diagnosed with spinocerebellar ataxia. It has been shown to improve physical capacity of the patient, slow the progression of the disease and limit the severity of the physical symptoms of the condition [25]. Furthermore, physical activity has been found to improve antioxidant capacity and reduction in prooxidant damage in patients with spinocerebellar ataxia [26]. It is therefore important, that green spaces are maintained, gyms and other facilities are created, and physical therapy is made available to this population so that the positive influence of physical activity can be accessed by this population.

2.7 Health condition

Non-communicable diseases account for more than half of the annual deaths in middle eastern countries [22]. The resultant public health advice has been targeted at reducing obesity through dietary and lifestyle changes to produce nutritional and general wellness. Despite the drive to improve dietary intake of complex carbohydrates, fruits and vegetables and reduce simple sugars, saturated fats and total cholesterol the rates of overweight and obesity continue to rise with a concordant increase in the Disability adjusted life years (DALY) [23]. Neurological disorders categorized as other account for approximately 2.5% of all neurological disorders between 1990–2015 and remains a significant concern especially in developed countries (**Figure 2**). Nevertheless, health condition remains and important

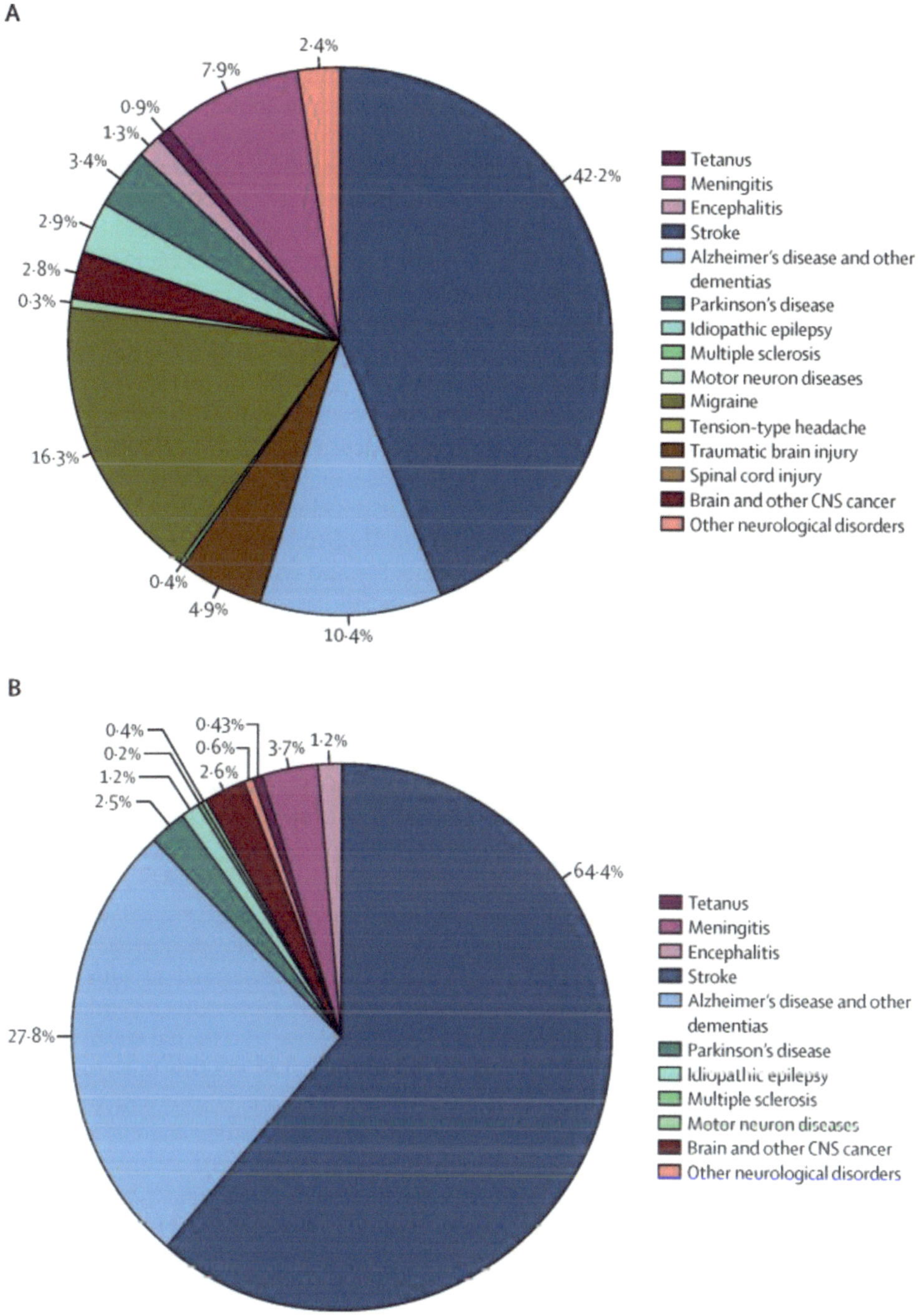

Figure 2.
The global burden of neurological disorders ([27], p. 258).

factor that influences dietary requirements and recommendations. In clients with neurological disorders especially spinocerebellar ataxia, there are several health conditions that impact on nutrition particularly requirements and dietary intake. Importantly the health conditions of these patients are also affected by nutritional status and intake. Individuals diagnosed with spinocerebellar ataxia experience, dysphagia, loss of lean body mass with weight loss, uncoordinated movement, micronutrient deficiencies including- niacin (Vitamin B_3), Tocopherol (Vitamin E) and thiamine (Vitamin B_1) as well as impaired fat metabolism and increased metabolism and prooxidant activity [3, 4, 14–16]. Dysphagia, uncoordinated movement, and loss of skeletal muscle mass may together create a challenge with feeding and limit dietary intake potentiating weight loss and reducing quality of life. Consequently, texture modification through thickening of food with caregiver support may help to treat swallowing difficulties and improve dietary intake. Limited muscle mass may be treated by introducing branched chain amino acids from supplements and complete proteins [28]. Micronutrient deficiencies constitute a health concern in spinocerebellar ataxia insomuch as they may influence negatively immune response, antioxidant capacity and energy metabolism ataxia [14–16]. It is therefore imperative that biochemical profile assessments are regularly conducted with a view to guide nutritional support. Increases in complete protein may supply adequate niacin levels, while thiamine levels can be improved from animal-based protein and tocopherol levels can be bolstered by consuming vegetable oils, green leafy vegetables and fortified cereals [29, 30]. Impaired fat metabolism is a critical concern in adults in general, and clients with spinocerebellar ataxia in particular, as this anomaly may lead to cardiovascular health risks including atherosclerosis and may also play a role in non-communicable disease development [6, 15]. To mitigate the negative health outcomes of impaired fat metabolism, caution needs to be taken with respect to meal preparation styles, limiting fry and trimming fats, and the selection of foods items [31]. Foods best suited in this case, should limit trans-fat, thereby reducing processed foods as well as increasing the intake of polyunsaturated fats from fish and nut oils while reducing saturated fats from red meats and animal fat. Finally, prooxidant activity in spinocerebellar ataxia can be managed through the reduction of processed foods, which are thought to have higher levels of prooxidant species and include foods with higher antioxidant capacity such as allium vegetables, fruits and a controlled amount of red wine [32]. Furthermore, when the immune status and antioxidant capacity of clients with spinocerebellar ataxia falls to suboptimal level, several nutritional approaches can be employed to improve these health statuses including supplementation and immunonutrition. Diet has been used to positively influence wellness through positive links with supplemental nutritional support, emotional wellness and immunonutrition. Supplemental nutrition includes the addition of a substance or product with the express goal of improving the intake of key micronutrients including vitamins and minerals [33]. This additional intake is aimed at improving nutritional status and wellness and has been a feature of the public health response in LMICs. It may also be employed in dietary options for clients who have low levels of micronutrients or those who are found to be clinically deficient, which is possible in clients with spinocerebellar ataxia. Supplemental nutrition may be formulated as tablets, pills, shakes and other products. Moreover, immunonutriton is a process or product of bolstering the immunity of individuals through the introduction of a targeted nutrients such as amino acids, especially essential and branched chain, essential poly unsaturated fatty acids, nucleotides, and antioxidants. It is particularly useful in reducing recovery time, improving quality of life and health of individuals who are immunosuppressed [21, 34]. This is another strategy that can be coupled with biochemical analysis to improve the immune status of the client when per os dietary support has not significantly improved antioxidant capacity, immune status, or micronutrient profile.

3. Summary and recommendations

Diet is associated with Quality of Life and Wellness. Several factors impact on the quality of dietary intake including social, physiological, and psychological issues. The dietary quality has important health outcomes ranging from impacts on Disability Life Years to an increased impact on disease burden, risk of concomitant diseases and impact of disease progression. Nevertheless, diet has been shown to improve body weight, muscle strength, immune capacity, disease progression, life expectancy, recovery, and general wellness especially in clients with spinocerebellar ataxia. Given the significance of diet in influencing the illness wellness continuum, public health officials are constantly challenged to improve the population outcomes using diet. The benefits of diet particularly its impact on improving the quality of life of clients with spinocerebellar ataxia, can be best achieved if portion control, nutrient density and meal planning were to be engaged in this population. Portion control addresses the concerns of caloric intake, through a general reduction in the size and amount of a meal at any single sitting and matches caloric requirements with intake goals [35]. This is associated with a strong positive linear relationship with weight maintenance and disease related quality of life. As energy balance is reached, caloric intake equilibrium is achieved, and weight maintenance is maintained even in high metabolic states. This strategy is particularly important as weight loss is mitigated and weight maintenance is achieved. Weight stabilization is an important factor in spinocerebellar ataxia and is an important determinant of disease progression. Nutrient density is a concept of increasing the range of nutrients consumed, particularly micronutrients, for the smallest value of calories [36, 37]. This allows for the increased functional activity of antioxidants, immune supportive micronutrients, and biological supportive nutrients [38]. The concordant impact on recovery, immune support, and reduction in prooxidant activity is important in wellness especially in clients diagnosed with spinocerebellar ataxia in view of the morbidity risk. Meal planning includes multiple principles that benefit overall dietary pattern through the improvement with calorie intake, through energy control, improving diversity and variety and instituting moderation. These result in planned meals that are better aligned with nutritional guidelines and associated with better health outcomes. Generally, these three principles of portion control, nutrient density and meal planning improve the metabolic profile of the individuals who consistently institute these practices, with improved Body Mass Index (BMI) values, more ideal body weight, healthier body fat and lipid profile with lower chronic disease risk profile. The benefits to be had from diet are best achieved with consistency, moderation and diligence and provide significant sustainable advantages to quality of life and wellness. In clients with neurological disorders, coordinated nutritional support and control are positively associated with better disease related quality of life through weight control, healthy micronutrient status and calorie control. It is essential that these activities are guided by appropriate biochemical and clinical tests and involve personalized and individualized strategies for the most beneficial impact. When instituted in spinocerebellar ataxia, dietary programmes involving principles of meal planning, nutrient density and energy balance redound to significant health outcomes such as weight maintenance, with slowed disease progression, improved immune status and healthy micronutrient. Therefore, a multi-team approach is recommended if the best health outcomes are to be achieved in spinocerebellar ataxia ensuring the involvement of the nutritionist/ dietician, the biochemist/ phlebotomist, physiotherapist, the neurologist and the general medical practitioner.

Author details

Donnette Alicia Wright* and Kadiann Peta-Gay Hewitt-Thompson
The University of the West Indies, Mona, Kingston, Jamaica

*Address all correspondence to: donnette.wright02@uwimona.edu.jm

References

[1] Klockgether, T., Mariotti, C., & Paulson, H. L. (2019). Spinocerebellar ataxia. Nature reviews Disease primers, 5(1), 1-21.

[2] Sullivan, R., Yau, W. Y., O'Connor, E., & Houlden, H. (2019). Spinocerebellar ataxia: an update. Journal of neurology, 266(2), 533-544.

[3] Cruz, M. M. S., Leite, C. D. M. B. A., Schieferdecker, M. E. M., Teive, H. A. G., Vieira, B. D., & Moro, A. (2019). Estimation of skeletal muscle mass in patients with spinocerebellar ataxia type 3 and 10. International Journal of Neuroscience, 129(7), 698-702.

[4] Rönnefarth, M., Hanisch, N., Brandt, A. U., Mähler, A., Endres, M., Paul, F., & Doss, S. (2020). Dysphagia Affecting Quality of Life in Cerebellar Ataxia—a Large Survey. The Cerebellum, 1-9.

[5] Wright, D. (2019). Nutrition and Hospital Mortality, Morbidity and Health Outcomes. In Strategies to Reduce Hospital Mortality in Lower and Middle Income Countries (LMICs) and Resource-Limited Settings. IntechOpen.

[6] Çekici, H., & Acar Tek, N. (2020). Determining energy requirement and evaluating energy expenditure in neurological diseases. Nutritional neuroscience, 23(7), 543-553.

[7] Kim S. (2014) World Health Organization Quality of Life (WHOQOL) Assessment. In: Michalos A.C. (eds) Encyclopedia of Quality of Life and Well-Being Research. Springer, Dordrecht. https://doi.org/10.1007/978-94-007-0753-5_3282.

[8] National Center for Chronic Disease Prevention and Health Promotion. (2018). Health Related Quality of Life (HRQOL). Retrieved from, https://www.cdc.gov/hrqol/concept.htm.

[9] Santos, L. R., Teive, H. A. G., Lopes Neto, F. D. N., Macedo, A. C. B. D., Mello, N. M. D., & Zonta, M. B. (2018). Quality of life in individuals with spinocerebellar ataxia type 10: a preliminary study. Arquivos de neuro-psiquiatria, 76(8), 527-533.

[10] Davis, T. (2019). What Is Well-Being? Definition, Types, and Well-Being Skills. Retrieved from, https://www.psychologytoday.com/intl/blog/click-here-happiness/201901/what is-well-being-definition-types-and-well-being-skills.

[11] Kabir, Miah & Islam. (2018). Factors influencing eating behavior and dietary intake among resident students in a public university in Bangladesh: A qualitative study. PLOS ONE. 13. e0198801. 10.1371/journal.pone.0198801.

[12] Wright, D., & Hewitt-Thompson, K. (2020). Nutritional Woes in a Pandemic: A Developing Country's Perspective. *International Journal of Innovative Science and Research* Technology, 5(4), 859-861.

[13] Diallo, A., Jacobi, H., Schmitz-Hübsch, T., Cook, A., Labrum, R., Durr, A., ... & Tezenas du Montcel, S. (2017). Body mass index decline is related to spinocerebellar ataxia disease progression. Movement disorders clinical practice, 4(5), 689-697.

[14] Camargo, S. M., Vuille-dit-Bille, R. N., Meier, C. F., & Verrey, F. (2020). ACE2 and gut amino acid transport. Clinical Science, 134(21), 2823-2833.

[15] Ko, C. W., Qu, J., Black, D. D., & Tso, P. (2020). Regulation of intestinal lipid metabolism: current concepts and relevance to disease. Nature Reviews Gastroenterology & Hepatology, 17(3), 169-183.

[16] Torres-Ramos, Y., Montoya-Estrada, A., Cisneros, B., Tercero-Pérez, K., León-Reyes, G., Leyva-García, N., ... & Magaña, J. J. (2018). Oxidative stress in spinocerebellar Ataxia type 7 is associated with disease severity. The Cerebellum, 17(5), 601-609.

[17] Fletcher, J. (2020). What is appetite?. Retrieved from,https://www.medicalnewstoday.com/articles/appetite

[18] Sarva, H., & Shanker, V. L. (2014). Treatment options in degenerative cerebellar ataxia: a systematic review. Movement disorders clinical practice, 1(4), 291-298.

[19] Jodhun, B. M., Pem, D., & Jeewon, R. (2016). A systematic review of factors affecting energy intake of adolescent girls. African Health Sciences, *16*(4), 910-922.

[20] van der Meij, B. S., Wijnhoven, H. A., Lee, J. S., Houston, D. K., Hue, T., Harris, T. B., Kritchevsky, S. B., Newman, A. B., & Visser, M. (2017). Poor appetite and dietary intake in community-dwelling older adults. Journal of the American Geriatrics Society, *65*(10), 2190-2197.

[21] Llauradó, G., Morris, H. J., Lebeque, Y., Venet, G., Fong, O., Marcos, J., Fontaine, R., Cos, P., & Bermúdez, R. C. (2016). Oral administration of an aqueous extract from the oyster mushroom Pleurotus ostreatus enhances the immunonutritional recovery of malnourished mice. Biomedicine & Pharmacotherapy, *83*, 1456-1463.

[22] Kilpi, F., Webber, L., Musaigner, A., Aitsi-Selmi, A., Marsh, T., Rtveladze, K., McPherson, K., & Brown, M. (2014). Alarming predictions for obesity and non-communicable diseases in the Middle East. Public health nutrition, *17*(5), 1078-1086.

[23] Kraemer, K., Cordaro, J., Fanzo, J., Gibney, M., Kennedy, E., Labrique, A., Steffen, J., & Eggersdorfer, M. (2016). Diet and non-communicable diseases: an urgent need for new paradigms. In *Good nutrition: Perspectives for the 21st century* (pp. 105-118). Karger Publishers.

[24] Shay, E., Khattak, A. J., & Wali, B. (2018). Walkability in the connected and automated vehicle era: a US perspective on research needs. Transportation research record, 2672(35), 118-128.

[25] Lanza, G., Casabona, J. A., Bellomo, M., Cantone, M., Fisicaro, F., Bella, R., ... & Bramanti, A. (2020). Update on intensive motor training in spinocerebellar ataxia: time to move a step forward?. Journal of International Medical Research, 48(2), 0300060519854626.

[26] Tercero-Pérez, K., Cortés, H., Torres-Ramos, Y., Rodríguez-Labrada, R., Cerecedo-Zapata, C. M., Hernández-Hernández, O., ... & Magaña, J. J. (2019). Effects of physical rehabilitation in patients with spinocerebellar ataxia type 7. The Cerebellum, 18(3), 397-405.

[27] Feigin, V.L., Vos, T., Nichols, E., Owolabi, M.O., Carroll, W. M., Dichgans, M., Deuschl, G., Parmar, P., Brainin, M & Murray, C. (2020). The global burden of neurological disorders: translating evidence into policy. The Lancet Neurology, 19 (3), 255-265.

[28] Ten Haaf, D. S., Eijsvogels, T. M., Bongers, C. C., Horstman, A. M., Timmers, S., de Groot, L. C., & Hopman, M. T. (2019). Protein supplementation improves lean body mass in physically active older adults: a randomized placebo-controlled trial. Journal of cachexia, sarcopenia and muscle, 10(2), 298-310.

[29] Çatak, J. (2019). Determination of niacin profiles in some animal and plant based foods by high performance

liquid chromatography: association with healthy nutrition. Journal of animal science and technology, 61(3), 138.

[30] Das Gupta, S., & Suh, N. (2016). Tocopherols in cancer: An update. Molecular nutrition & food research, 60(6), 1354-1363.

[31] Julibert, A., del Mar Bibiloni, M., & Tur, J. A. (2019). Dietary fat intake and metabolic syndrome in adults: a systematic review. Nutrition, Metabolism and Cardiovascular Diseases, 29(9), 887-905.

[32] Rodriguez-Casado, A. (2016). The health potential of fruits and vegetables phytochemicals: notable examples. Critical Reviews in Food Science and Nutrition, 56(7), 1097-1107.

[33] Raiten, D. J., Allen, L. H., Slavin, J. L., Mitloehner, F. M., Thoma, G. J., Haggerty, P. A., & Finley, J. W. (2020). Understanding the intersection of climate/environmental change, health, agriculture and improved nutrition: a case study on micronutrient nutrition and animal source foods. *Current Developments in Nutrition*.

[34] Celiberto, L. S., Graef, F. A., Healey, G. R., Bosman, E. S., Jacobson, K., Sly, L. M., & Vallance, B. A. (2018). Inflammatory bowel disease and immunonutrition: novel therapeutic approaches through modulation of diet and the gut microbiome. Immunology, *155*(1), 36-52.

[35] Rolls, B. J. (2018). The role of portion size, energy density, and variety in obesity and weight management. Handbook of obesity treatment, 93-104.

[36] Bouis, H. E., & Welch, R. M. (2010). Biofortification—a sustainable agricultural strategy for reducing micronutrient malnutrition in the global south. *Crop Science*, *50*, S-20-S-32.

[37] Drewnowski, A. (2005). Concept of a nutritious food: toward a nutrient density score. The American Journal of Clinical Nutrition, *82*(4), 721-732.

[38] Lockyer, S., Cade, J., Darmon, N., Flynn, M., Gatenby, S., Govindji, A., Quick, B., Raats, M., Rayner, M., & Sokolović, M. (2020). Proceedings of a roundtable event 'Is communicating the concept of nutrient density important?'. Nutrition Bulletin, *45*(1), 74-97.

Section 2

Classification: Subtypes and Symptoms

Chapter 3

International Classification of Functioning, Health and Disability (ICF) Conceptual Approach towards Spinocerebellar Ataxia

Kevin Triangto, Steven Setiono and Herdiman Bernard Purba

Abstract

Spinocerebellar Ataxia (SCA) is an autosomal dominant disease with progressive decline towards functional capacity. Although studies had shown that there are various SCA types, physical medicine and rehabilitation approach would focus mostly on functional aspects in each individuals. Analysis through International Classification of Functioning, Disability, and Health would assist clinicians to identify activity and participation aspects of SCA, mostly revolves around mobility function. Good correlation of mobility with quality of life was also reported, and thus it is only natural that this becomes the main focus of rehabilitative intervention. Approximately one hour physical exercise session focusing on postural control and balance was proven to be effective in improving disease related measurement tool, functional capacity, and quality of life. These benefits could be improved through newer therapies such as exercise games and virtual reality, virtually creates a rapidly changing environment, thus providing training through anticipatory actions. It is speculated that neuroplasticity through self-recognition of errors are the main physiology of recovery in SCA. Finally, it could be seen that rehabilitation intervention remains to be a cornerstone in current ataxia therapy, with goals of achieving exercise gains while alleviating the natural functional decline of the disease.

Keywords: Spinocerebellar Ataxia, physical medicine, rehabilitation, balance exercise, neuroplasticity

1. Introduction

Spinocerebellar Ataxia (SCA) is well known to be an autosomal dominant progressive disease that significantly affect quality of life [1]. Despite the many types of SCA based on genetic code variations, which are reflected in varying severity of symptoms, studies have shown that balance problem remained to be the mainstay reason in quality of life reductions [2]. Due to the appearance of all these symptoms, it is still a challenge in prioritizing problems to be managed in order to provide the best impact. One common language that is generally used as a functioning concept in physical medicine and rehabilitation field, is known as the International Classification of Functioning, Disability, and Health (ICF) concept [3]. Several investigations had shown that utilizing this concept in rehabilitation would substantially enhance success due to better prioritization of problems. Although rehabilitation had been demonstrated to be a cornerstone in ataxia therapy, reports about ICF in SCA rehabilitation is still very much lacking [4].

While rehabilitation could alleviate several symptoms of SCA, many concerned if these therapies could match the speed of natural progression in this disease [4, 5]. As a general overview of rehabilitation interventions, it could be majorly divided into technique based rehabilitation exercises, and the utilization of modalities [2, 6, 7]. Exercises are then more specifically classified to each professionals in the rehabilitation team, namely physiotherapist, occupational therapist, and speech therapist. Each of the rehabilitation team play an essential part towards the holistic care of SCA subjects, and hence has to be well apprehended. On the other hand, modern therapy modalities have emerged as adjuncts to conventional therapy [8, 9]. These newer modalities are targeted to improve neuroplasticity in SCA subjects as the residual brain potential towards better functioning [10]. Therefore, this chapter is dedicated to review the comprehensive management of SCA from the physical medicine and rehabilitation point of view.

2. International classification of functioning, disability and health (ICF) concept on spinocerebellar ataxia

Over the years there seem to be growing evidence on the language of physical medicine and rehabilitation, especially in defining disability and its impact to both the individual and the society they live. The most recent terminology utilizes the International Classification of Functioning, Disability and Health (ICF) concept [3]. The ICF concept is a supplement of the 10th revision of International Statistical Classification of Diseases and Related Health Problems by World Health Organization (ICD X), that comprehensively describes an individual's health condition while still accounting their performance in community [3]. This concept could then ease physiatrists in creating both treatment goals and therapy focus which are tailor made for the individual.

Utilizing ICF in the daily practice requires the use of several core sets which are specified for the disease, but this however has been a challenge as not all diseases have their specific core sets published. As SCA have no specific core set yet, it is then recommended for physiatrist to adapt to an existing core set which has similar properties, and chronic stroke core set would seem most fitting to an ongoing central neurological disorder [11]. Aside from utilizing the core set, it is important to focus on some components of the ICF concept that could become the focus of the treatment plan, emphasizing on setting achievable goals by using several measuring tools.

In a glance it could be seen that the ICF concept starts with describing the body structure and body function after stating the diagnosis [3]. Afterwards, activity and participation should be listed as to describe the individuals' challenges in performing activity of daily living or even in the community level [3]. The next subsection of ICF involves description of environmental factors that would affect the individual, be it from physical environment or the community they are involved in [3]. Last but not least, personal factors should be addressed as well, knowing that adherence and motivation would affect the success of a rehabilitation program.

2.1 Body structure and body function

The focus of body structure in spinocerebellar ataxia is obviously the cerebellum, in the spinocerebellum (center) portion. It is known that the spinocerebellum gathers a large volume of sensory information from the peripheral organs, as well as relaying information from the motor cortex [12, 13]. Etiologically this is caused by autosomal dominant mutation on the SCA gene, and this would disrupt the connection between multiple layers of cerebellum [1]. Prior studies had shown that severity of symptoms would correlate to the cerebellar areas involvement, and differs between various types of SCA [2, 7, 14]. Ultimately these changes result in functional disturbances as well as learning difficulties [15, 16].

One of the main body function disorders in SCA that should be addressed is balance and postural control [9, 17]. Consistently studies had shown that balance is disturbed both during static and dynamic, hence implies difficulty in performing effective gait, and maintaining standing position [9, 18, 19]. Since cerebellum also becomes a relay center for agonist and antagonistic complimentary contractions, it is natural to see that spinocerebellum lesion would affect effective voluntary muscle contractions, which could also present as central hypotonia [4, 6]. As discussed earlier, learning difficulties in SCA would span its impact from impaired conditional skill learning, up until reduced ability in adapting changes from environment [15, 16]. All these errors in cerebellar signaling would also result in poor coordination, as there are several mismatches in relaying sensory information to produce an effective motor response, as well as poor intra-limb coordination in spinocerebellum damage [20, 21]. Limited study are available in exploration of autonomic function disorder, and it was reported that overactive bladder is most commonly seen in SCA 2 [22]. Therefore, despite the local extent of damage in body structure, the functional impact is notoriously destructive.

2.2 Activity and participation

Having the body function described, it could be inferred that there would be a wide range of activity and participation disorders in SCA patients. One of the most reported problem in activity would be gait efficacy, as the lesion will interfere limb advancing patterns, as well as poor alternative terrain adaptability [8, 19]. Despite the inferior quality of life in motor control, the patients could still communicate as there are supposedly no barrier in this [23]. Even so, several studies revealed that cognitive impairments are found in SCA with varying severity [15, 16]. A number of studies have also reported that difficulty in verbal memory, learning, and fluency are commonly seen [16, 24]. These cognitive disorders would sum into a restriction in several community participation, but motor abilities still remained to inflict the most significant effect to quality of life in SCA [25]. Reports have mentioned the involvement of visuospatial and executive functioning abilities being reduced in SCA3, as it may correlate with reduced cerebellar perfusion [16]. Learning abilities in particular, were consistently shown to be retained in prodromal SCA2, as neural plasticity may still be prominent with Brain Derived Neurotrophic Factor playing its role, and other parts of the brain compensating for the functional deficit [15]. These evidences of preserved learning abilities in progressive disorders, must be recognized in the highest priority, knowing it would be the key to efficient rehabilitation for SCA cases [26–28].

2.3 Environmental and personal factors

The main environmental factor issues that was addressed for SCA is the difficulty to walk on varying level terrains [13, 29, 30]. It should be remembered that stable walking in varying level terrains require several functions ranging from cognition, vision, limb control, and balance. Severe fatigue was also seen in 69% of SCA patients, and thus different SCA types would result in different lesion focus and function disorder [31]. Moreover, since learning abilities are also compromised, a combination of these symptoms would ultimately result in terrain adaptation barriers [1, 4]. These should be identified in each patients, and correlated to their living environment in order to formulate an effective intervention.

Depression were consistently reported in several studies on SCA, and this could correlate significantly with quality of life [22, 30]. As mentioned previously that mobility is the main concern, depression levels were also seen lower in those subjects with better mobility [6, 25]. Even when other causes of depression may revolve around memory and learning ability disorders, most SCA subjects would have learning difficulty in limb control, which becomes a vicious cycle and a hazard for them to perform well in mobile activities of daily living [5]. Therefore, early detection of depression is important, especially in the personal factors subsection of ICF.

Although physical medicine and rehabilitation approach to SCA might differ between studies, it's observable that the main focus is always towards body function, activity and participation. This focus is generally uncommon to be seen in the published studies, since most of these studies would focus on exploring various types of SCA, such as SCA1, SCA2, SCA3, SCA6 and SCA7 that are commonly found in the community [1, 7, 14, 27]. Shortly put, rehabilitative approach to SCA would place its greatest weigh on identifying disorders of body function through physical examination, rather than determining the SCA type through genetic testing [6]. In any case, each individual must receive tailor made interventions even when they are in the same SCA type.

3. Rehabilitation strategies for spinocerebellar ataxia

In response to the stated functional problems, various rehabilitation strategies have been implemented and studied over the years [2, 6, 7]. Surely mobility and balance interventions have been one of the main focus in SCA studies, however through time, studies have widened their range of focus into endurance, cognition, and speech [30]. Rehabilitation strategies may be a combination of several mode of interventions, such as exercise, physical modality, and sensory stimulation [9, 14, 27].

Comprehensive examination is required prior to these interventions, as each patients should receive tailormade intervention, and thus not all of these strategies are administered to all patients. Through utilization of ICF conceptual analysis, then clinicians should focus on body function problems identified in SCA patients, as shown on **Table 1** that depicts the common functional problems seen in SCA subtypes. This subsection will discuss these strategies in detail to give an overview of what is being studied in the published studies.

3.1 Physiotherapy interventions

Majority of the published studies have mentioned how physiotherapy plays a big role in mobility interventions of SCA patients, be it through conventional therapy or through exergames and virtual reality [9]. Since physiotherapy intervention is primarily focused on achieving better gait control, it would naturally revolve on improving balance, strength, endurance, and posture simultaneously [18, 27]. This finding has resulted into a more focused exercise sessions in the recent studies, aiming mainly on trunk balance, as these would be positively reflected in significant improvement of Scale for the Assessment and Rating of Ataxia (SARA) score [19, 38].

Although there are no published guidelines on SCA mobility exercise, several published studies from Cuban Centre for the Research and Rehabilitation

No	Function	SCA Type
1	Sensory and Motor Cortex [13]	6
2	Ataxia & Cognition [15]	2
3	Falls, Balance Impairment, & Functional Mobility [29]	1, 2, 3, 6
4	Non-motor & Extracerebellar [22]	2
5	Cognitive [24]	6
6	Action perception cerebellar recruitment [26]	6
7	Dystonia [32]	1, 2, 3, 6
8	Cognitive & Socio-cognitive [16]	1, 2, 3, 6, 7
9	Clinical & Genetic of Brain MRI Changes [33]	1, 2
10	Motor & Cognitive – brain volume [34]	7
11	Autonomic Function [35]	2
12	Non ataxic manifestations [36]	2
13	Dysphagia [37]	3, 6

Table 1.
Spinocerebellar functional problems in common SCA types.

of Hereditary Ataxia (CIRAH) had effectively shown the benefits of intensive neurorehabilitation as they have conducted [18, 27]. The whole therapy lasted for four hours per day, five days per week, lasting for 12 weeks in total, hence to the authors' knowledge, this is the longest exercise duration seen per day. Daily tasks include both physiotherapy and occupational therapy interventions, with several breaks in between to restore both energy and training focus. It could be resumed that majority of the exercises given in CIRAH's daily tasks include static balance improvement, and positional changes, all to improve trunk control and complement daily living tasks being trained by occupational therapists. Another important component that should be noted is the coordination exercises, which trains intra-limb coordination [18, 27]. These sets of exercises had proven to be very effective in improving cerebellar symptoms, as reflected in constant improvement of SARA scores of both SCA subjects in early prodromal stage and SCA2 diagnosed 11 years mean post onset [18, 27].

Other studies had utilized shorter sessions as compared to the CIRAH neurorehabilitation schedule, but all these had shown significant improvement of SARA scores. One such study reported that partial Body Weight Supported Treadmill Training could improve balance significantly, and general positive trend in improving mobility, endurance, and quality of life [19]. It could be possible that these studies alike are more focused on providing intervention in trunk control, which is parallel to the fact that trunk ataxia has better prognosis as compared to limb incoordination in SCA. Another concern lies that there are controversies in the outcome measurement of SARA scores, as they are very sensitive in detecting cerebellar symptoms, but not for extracerebellar symptoms. Despite those controversies, SARA scores could still be utilized as it correlates closely to functional abilities, and thus would pertain to be an effective evaluation tool in SCA studies.

Additionally, consistent evidence revealed that trunk ataxia could have better rehabilitation prognosis as compared to limb ataxia [8, 39]. The main problem persists that the rate of degeneration at every year must be matched with beneficial gains from exercise, and thus effective regimens would be the primary choice as a rehabilitation goal. The natural progression of SARA score in SCA is noted to be

0.6 to 2.5 points per year, whereas it was shown in most studies how training would effectively reduce SARA at least by one point, displaying clinical importance of these interventions [5].

3.2 Virtual reality and exercise games

It could be acknowledged that maintaining the provided gains from exercise is of importance in degenerative disorder [2, 6]. Several recent studies had revealed how exergames (exercise games) and immersive virtual reality would be able to fill up this shortfall in conventional therapy [8, 9]. Exergames here are considered adjuvant to the traditional physiotherapy, and could never replace their roles in ataxia rehabilitation [9]. An important feature in exergames that should be highlighted, is the fact that there are rapidly changing environment, thus demands an accurate anticipation from the ataxic cases, providing excellent gains to the sensorimotor system [9]. These anticipation were shown to correlate with real life situations, and could effectively maintain exercise effects throughout longer period [8, 9].

Proper choosing of modalities would benefit SCA subjects in different stages, where early stages could follow high demand competitive sporting exergames such as ping-pong, badminton and squash [8]. These exergames and virtual reality should be performed on elastic carpet, as it's shown to give additional benefits in improving coordination and postural control through proprioceptive feedback. More severe ataxia would not allow them to play on competitive exergames, and would obtain greater advantage from good postural control. Games such as tightrope walk, which requires the user to maintain a specific position while still advancing forward, had been reported to effectively enhance both static and dynamic balance [8]. On the other hand, mild to moderate stages would benefit from conventional coordinative physiotherapy and severe stages though have no clear guidelines yet [9]. Hence it's shown how exergames would play its best role in early stages, and also to maintain the gains accrued from conventional physiotherapy. As stated previously that studies had shown how mobility learning mechanisms may still be preserved in SCA cases, these newer therapies would then be targeted to hone these adaptive skills and apply them to their daily situations.

3.3 Trunk and intra-limb control

While many studies had shown how trunk control could have many exercise options, improving limb control has been shown as a big challenge in SCA subjects. It was also reported that good intra limb control is best seen in walking analysis, observing their coordination in performing effective transition from single and double leg stance [19]. Several studies had shown that static cycling would be an effective intervention to improve intra limb control [20, 21]. A controlled trial comprising of four week long cycling exercise was reported to restore the ability in modulating H-reflex inhibition, and is also correlated with better functional performances [40]. Although the impact was not as major as their healthy control counterpart, it could be seen that cycling would present itself as a potential exercise option for improving coordination in SCA subjects [40]. Added effects of endurance and strength gains through stationary cycling has also been reported, especially in mobility disorder patients such as cerebral palsy [41].

Postural exercise approach are generally based on "re-learning" strategies of destabilizing responses, that anticipatory movements are trained in various environments, as well as honing of sensorimotor reflexes in the light of preserved plasticity [9, 13]. Postural instability would also lead to chronic low back pain, and thus stretching must also be given in order to alleviate these before and after training sessions [9]. One voxel based study had shown 2 weeks of postural training would lead to improvement of balance, which was maintained for 3 months after training. Additionally, gray matter volume would also increase, and interestingly it is on the non-affected areas, meaning to say that targeted plasticity lies in the cerebral areas to compensate their cerebellar loss [28]. The study had mentioned that dorsal premotor cortex obtained the most compelling change, as they project to primary motor cortex and cerebellum, all of which are involved in movement planning and motor learning. Both patients and controls demonstrated an increase in gray matter volume in temporal association areas, this may be due to the requirement of performing sequential actions, which would in turn stimulates procedural memories in both hippocampus and basal ganglia. Cerebellar changes post exercise are not seen in cerebellar degenerative disorders as expected, but is significantly seen in healthy controls, with parallel increase in visuospatial and temporal inputs. These would then show how interventions towards premotor cortex growth should be the main goal of exercise in SCA subjects in preserving mobility [28].

3.4 Occupational therapy interventions

Besides physiotherapy interventions, occupational therapy is another important modality within the attempts of improving quality of life in SCA subjects [9, 42]. As mentioned previously, occupational therapy is usually incorporated with physiotherapy courses [18]. In the big picture, they should be given after warm up stretches to obtain better postural control during the specific exercises. In the published studies, mainly occupational therapy intervention would have a one hour duration, and this addition have been proven effective in improving both SARA and Functional Independence Measure (FIM) scores. The program itself consists of basic activity of daily living exercises, which are essentially a part of the FIM and Barthel Index Scoring sheet. Some of the examples include dressing activities such as tying shoelaces, buttoning shirts; tabletop instrumental activities for instance inserting sewing needles, drawing, cutting paper figures, using keyboards; and finally communication activities like reading texts out loud, commenting and interpreting verbal and textual information [18].

Despite the promising effects, studies focusing on occupational therapy as an individual therapy is still lacking due to the progressive nature of the disease, thus could only be shown as an additive effect to the proven effective physiotherapy. A study had shown that occupational therapy would improve Hamilton scores for depression in SCA3, and this improvement was independent from its confounders [42]. So far there are no studies yet on occupational therapy being a home program, but it could be speculated that more frequent practices would eventually trigger better quality synapses in the brain, leading to a more superior functional improvement. Therefore, aside from improving the functional abilities, it could also be inferred that occupational therapy would enhance self-confidence, alleviates depressive mood, and thus forecasts better participation [9, 42].

3.5 Speech therapy interventions

In order to fully complement the comprehensive care of SCA patients, speech and language pathology should be addressed to achieve well-being [23]. However, there are very few studies that discusses this, since only few types of ataxia that has bulbar involvement and thus results in dysphagia due to excess salivation [43]. A study had shown and compared how dysphagia is more severe in SCA3, whereas mild dysphagia is seen in SCA6 [37]. Possible treatment options would depend on related problems, but mostly rehabilitation targets is to increase willingness and independence [23, 43]. At the same time, swallowing exercise would also aim in cueing patients to gain self-recognition in their swallowing process, thus triggering anticipatory self-evaluation [23, 43]. Since cognition is also an identified problem in SCA, this could also be identified by the speech and language pathologist, and self-corrections cueing prove to be effective [23]. In a more severe cases, safe swallowing practice along with appropriate dietary modification may be done in order to prevent aspiration [23]. Despite the scarcity of studies, a Cochrane review on speech disorder treatment for hereditary ataxia revealed that all the rehabilitative interventions have been reported as safe, and hence should be recommended in the comprehensive care [43].

3.6 Neuroplasticity and therapy duration

Clinicians should always remember that neuroplasticity plays a big role in alleviating SCA cerebellar signs, as proven in SCA2 subjects [10]. Unfortunately, there are still no reported significant effect on non-ataxia signs [28]. It also appears that SCA2 subjects may have more progressive disorders, and thus 24 weeks of therapy was suggested, whereas for other types such as SCA6 and SCA31, 4 weeks of training may already show better SARA score improvements [27]. Thus, the extent of affected area in the cerebellum would correlate directly to the progressiveness, hence would warrant different sets of rehabilitation strategy. Recognizing the neuroplasticity potential of SCA individuals would assist clinicians in identifying therapy focus, as well as motivating patients and family members to improve exercise adherence.

3.7 Essential points in rehabilitation strategies

Although there is no general guideline on this, rehabilitation strategies would adhere to functional disorder basis, that each strategy is given only when the disorder is identified [1, 6, 9]. Due to the progressive nature of the disease though, it is also plausible to administer the intervention even when the disorder have not emerge, knowing the fact that it may alleviate functional deterioration in the future. Two things that should be remembered are that fatigue may be one of the limitation in performing all the available strategies, and secondly, maintenance in quality of life must always be upheld [30]. Despite not many studies focused on quality of life, clinical experiences showed that progressive disease rehabilitation interventions should emphasize on giving life to the rest of the years, rather than adding years to the remaining life.

4. Rehabilitation goals and expected outcome measures in spinocerebellar ataxia

Aligned with their natural progression of disease, rehabilitation goals in degenerative ataxias would differ significantly from acquired ataxias. It was shown that acquired ataxias such as in stroke cases, would come with focal ischemia, ergo a better prognosis as compared to the diffuse lesion in SCA [1, 44]. Additionally, the degenerative process of SCA is of the highest concern, therefore it must be addressed and evaluated with valid measuring tools. Several subjects that were focused in prior studies include functional abilities, mobility function, balance, endurance, and quality of life [30].

4.1 Disease related tools

Ataxia specific tools such as SARA and Inventory of Non-Ataxia Symptoms (INAS) are most commonly utilized in many studies [45, 46]. The SARA score is designed to assess cerebellar symptoms semiquantitatively, and exclusively only SCA subjects were tested during the validation process. The SARA score ranges from 0 to 40, higher number showing more severe ataxia, the values then reflect eight physical examination items each with specific numeric scores. Physical examination of gait, stationary standing, and sitting position are observed, with a cut off of maintaining 10 second stationary position without difficulty as sufficient. One common bulbar component of SCA being speech production is also evaluated, and will be scored worst if the subject could only do unintelligible speech during normal conversation. Last but not least, performance of coordination tests namely finger chase, nose to finger test, dysdiadochokinesia, and heel shin test are graded with a score of 4 as the worst performance. As could be seen in these scored items, all of these are included in the general rehabilitation examination of cerebellar symptoms, and therefore this score is very much applicable in daily practice. Consistently it was shown that SARA score would correlate closely to symptom severity, and thus could be practically used to evaluate the efficacy of rehabilitation program [45].

With that being said, the main limitation of SARA would be that other scorings are required in the light of addressing extracerebellar symptoms. Therefore, the same research group had devised INAS score which could quantify the presence and severity of non-ataxia neurological symptoms [46]. The inventory consists of 30 items that is divided into two main section, the first spans widely from addressing cerebellar oculomotor signs, spinal reflexes, upper and lower motor neuron signs through physical examination. The second section on the other hand, lists the possible symptoms that the patient might bring about, such as double vision, dysphagia, urinary dysfunction, cognitive impairment, and other related findings that have not been listed. Similarly, the INAS scoring was also validated by utilizing SCA subjects with varying types, namely SCA1, SCA2, SCA3, and SCA6. Among these SCA types, it was reported that SCA1 and SCA2 presents extracerebellar symptoms along with the baseline ataxia, thus they are good candidates for the INAS, while SCA6 being purely cerebellar would play its role as control. The summation of the score is called INAS count, in which they have concluded that both INAS and INAS count shows good reproducibility, but unsatisfactory responsiveness over extended period due to the wide variation of measurement [46]. However it was clearly shown that INAS is an excellent supplement to the SARA score for SCA subjects.

4.2 Functional measurement tools

Other studies had also shown that in very early ataxia stages, both SARA and INAS are ineffective in prodromal stage [18]. Functional test alternatives such as tandem gait for 5 meter test was suggested to be used, as it is very sensitive to changes post rehabilitation [18]. The tandem gait itself is a complex task which may not be performed well by all SCA subjects, therefore traditional balance assessments such as Berg Balance Scale (BBS) [17, 25, 44]. The BBS consist of 14 item list, with an ordinal scale of 0 to 4, higher number meaning better balance function. The main categories in the item list revolves around maintenance of stationary position, transfer, and change of position while performing simple activities. Summation of all the scores for less than 45 would indicate greater risks of falling [47]. In cases that the BBS is not used in total, the components could also be used individually to monitor a specific progression within therapy evaluation.

Another study had also utilized the timed up and go (TUG) test to evaluate balance and function in degenerative ataxia subjects [20, 21]. In several rehabilitation trials, TUG test are well preferred due to their ease of examination, quantification of results in seconds, and finally their best representation to daily living tasks. However in cases of SCA, probably the complete TUG test might not always be performable due to high risk of fall. Several studies had also utilized expanded TUG test, which divides the full TUG test into segments measured by milliseconds, namely sit to stand, gait 1, turning, gait 2, and stand to sit [48, 49]. By separating these components, physiatrists would have a better view on which component are hindering the subject in achieving good TUG performance, and at the same time, would be able to assess improvements more accurately. Although the expanded TUG have not been utilized in SCA studies, it has been commonly used in other chronic neurological cases such as stroke, and hence should be recommended for future studies on degenerative ataxia [48].

Aside from TUG test, a more comprehensive functional test tool such as functional independence measure (FIM) are commonly used in SCA studies [25]. The utilization of FIM had expanded the view on functional activities and illustrate their level of independence in those activities. The FIM tool comprise of several components such as bowel, bladder control, transfer, locomotion, social participation, communication and also self-care activities [50, 51]. These components will then be graded from 1 to 7, when value of 6 and above shows complete dependence, scores 3 to 5 shows moderate dependence, and lastly below 3 shows full dependence. Therefore, this tool would be best used when the subjects are not fully independent, and other individuals such as caregivers are involved. Naturally FIM would have a ceiling effect when the patient is fully independent, and there are no additional scoring for the performance quality.

In SCA subjects it was reported that reduction of 1 point in FIM score would be significantly reflected in 4.49 point decrease in the physical functioning of Short Form 36 (SF-36) score [25]. In the light of SF-36, it is the most commonly used tool to assess quality of life in SCA subjects. As the name implies, this tool has 36 questions which covers eight domains of health, for instance limitations in physical activities, social activities, role function, pain, emotional problem, mental health, fatigue, and finally general health perceptions [52]. Various ordinal options in each questions should firstly be calculated through a formula to obtain domain scores. This finding then reveals how FIM could also be used to assess overtime changes that would complement the changes in other ataxia specific tools, in which better mobility correlates with greater quality of life [25, 53].

4.3 Fatigue and endurance measurement tools

In relationship to quality of life, fatigue is pretty much prevalent and thus is essential to note. Aside from SF-36 that touches on the fatigue concept, the fatigue severity scale (FSS) is a specific 9 item scale which measures fatigue in a 1 to 7 scale, 7 being strongly agree with the fatigue item being stated [31]. Accomplishing the FSS requires only 5 minutes, but the questions would not accurately direct the underlying functional disorder beneath, especially in chronic cases where fatigue is evident. Therefore, both cardiovascular and respiratory specific tools must be administered separately in order to evaluate through time. There are a selected number of studies that discuss the changes of cardiorespiratory attributes through evaluation of maximum oxygen consumption (VO2 max), six minute walk test (6MWT), peak expiratory flow (PEF), and maximum inspiratory pressure (MIP) [21, 38, 54].

Evaluation of VO2 max is done by performing ramped ergometer exercise stress testing, while 6MWT could be performed with assistance if the subjects are unable to [21]. With all these limitations, it could be possible that evaluation of cardiovascular function will not be optimal owing to the natural progression of the disease and obstacles in maintaining stationary position. On the contrary, respiratory function has shorter examination time, allowing better examination compliance [54]. A recent study had shown how examination of both PEF and MIP are safe to be performed in SCA2 subjects, when better respiratory function seemed to correlate well with Activity of Daily Living scales, and ataxia specific SARA scales [54]. Additionally, the study had also reported that one third of the subjects complained of dyspnea, with interpretation of restrictive pulmonary disease. It is speculated that the restriction may be caused by the lack of coordination of the respiratory muscles, ultimately resulting in reduced chest expansion [54]. On the other point of view, postural control exercises would be able to improve diaphragmatic excursion, and thus provide attempts in correcting respiratory dysfunction [55–57]. Therefore, it is only possible that physiotherapy interventions to manage ataxia related symptoms also alleviate respiratory symptoms, thus very mild respiratory dysfunction that could be reported.

5. Conclusion

Being a progressive degenerative disease, physical medicine and rehabilitation have an important role in alleviating symptoms as well as improving quality of life in Spinocerebellar Ataxia [4]. Initial analysis of SCA begins with identifying the ICF concept, in which body structure being cerebellum, and several body function problems such as postural control and intra-limb control should firstly be addressed [8]. These underlying disorders would lead to below par daily living performance, further leading to restriction in participation, and might also result in depression [25, 30]. Nevertheless it should be remembered that there is a natural progression of functional decline, which is unavoidable in SCA [1]. Therefore, rehabilitation goals are generally focused in maintaining functional capacity, as well as improving social participation and quality of life [4].

Achieving the aforementioned rehabilitation goals could be done through several interventions, but it was shown that physiotherapy exercise sessions focused in improving posture, balance, and gait had proven to be the most effective. Duration of session generally lasts for 1 hour or more, but it should be preceded with stretching to ease pain and provide better proprioceptive feedback [18]. In order to enhance retaining of the exercise gains, proper choices of virtual reality and exergames could be done [8, 9]. Most studies have also incorporated occupational therapy that rehearses daily living activities, and it's seen to correlate well with quality of life [42]. Simultaneously, speech therapy would also play its role in SCA by managing communication and swallowing disorders that are present in several types of SCA [43]. Several valid outcome measuring tools have been shown effective to monitor changes over time, and it should be remembered that these measures could assess specific components that are being trained [22, 30]. In conclusion, effective rehabilitation approach should comprise of all the previously mentioned components, while always being validated by specific outcome measure tools. In addition to that, further studies should devise a guideline for general rehabilitation of SCA through validated trials.

Conflict of interest

The authors declare no conflict of interest.

Thanks

The corresponding author would like to mention a note of thanks to the ever-supporting wife, Gisca Meiviana, for all her constant encouragement during the process of authoring this book chapter, and for being an amazing life partner throughout.

Author details

Kevin Triangto[1*], Steven Setiono[2] and Herdiman Bernard Purba[2]

1 Cardiac Prevention and Rehabilitation Department, National Cardiovascular Center Harapan Kita, West Jakarta, Indonesia

2 Physical Medicine and Rehabilitation Department, Cipto Mangunkusumo Hospital University of Indonesia, Central Jakarta, Indonesia

*Address all correspondence to: kevintriangto14@gmail.com

References

[1] Klockgether T, Mariotti C, Paulson HL. Spinocerebellar ataxia. Nat Rev Dis Prim. 2019 Apr;5(1):24.

[2] Sullivan R, Yau WY, O'Connor E, Houlden H. Spinocerebellar ataxia: an update. J Neurol. 2019 Feb;266(2):533-44.

[3] WHO. ICF: International Classification of Functioning, Disability and Health. Geneva: World Health Organization; 2001.

[4] He M, Zhang H-N, Tang Z-C, Gao S-G. Balance and coordination training for patients with genetic degenerative ataxia: a systematic review. J Neurol. 2020 Jun;

[5] Barbuto S, Kuo S-H, Stein J. Investigating the Clinical Significance and Research Discrepancies of Balance Training in Degenerative Cerebellar Disease: A Systematic Review. Am J Phys Med Rehabil. 2020 Nov;99(11):989-98.

[6] Kelly G, Shanley J. Rehabilitation of ataxic gait following cerebellar lesions: Applying theory to practice. Physiother Theory Pract. 2016 Aug;32(6):430-7.

[7] Miyai I. Challenge of neurorehabilitation for cerebellar degenerative diseases. Cerebellum. 2012 Jun;11(2):436-7.

[8] Synofzik M, Ilg W. Motor training in degenerative spinocerebellar disease: ataxia-specific improvements by intensive physiotherapy and exergames. Biomed Res Int. 2014;2014:583507.

[9] Lanza G, Casabona JA, Bellomo M, Cantone M, Fisicaro F, Bella R, et al. Update on intensive motor training in spinocerebellar ataxia: time to move a step forward? J Int Med Res. 2020 Feb;48(2):300060519854626.

[10] Matsugi A, Kikuchi Y, Kaneko K, Seko Y, Odagaki M. Cerebellar transcranial magnetic stimulation facilitates excitability of spinal reflex, but does not affect cerebellar inhibition and facilitation in spinocerebellar ataxia. Neuroreport. 2018 Jul;29(10):808-13.

[11] Geyh S, Cieza A, Schouten J, Dickson H, Frommelt P, Omar Z, et al. ICF Core Sets for stroke. J Rehabil Med. 2004;36(SUPPL. 44):135-41.

[12] Mtui E, Gruener G, Dockery P. Cerebellum. In: Mtui E, Gruener G, Dockery P, editors. Fitzgerald's Clinical Neuroanatomy and Neuroscience. 7th ed. Philadelphia (PA): ELSEVIER; 2016. p. 243-52.

[13] Kang N, Christou EA, Burciu RG, Chung JW, DeSimone JC, Ofori E, et al. Sensory and motor cortex function contributes to symptom severity in spinocerebellar ataxia type 6. Brain Struct Funct. 2017 Mar;222(2):1039-52.

[14] Tercero-Pérez K, Cortés H, Torres-Ramos Y, Rodríguez-Labrada R, Cerecedo-Zapata CM, Hernández-Hernández O, et al. Effects of Physical Rehabilitation in Patients with Spinocerebellar Ataxia Type 7. Cerebellum. 2019 Jun;18(3):397-405.

[15] Gigante AF, Lelli G, Romano R, Pellicciari R, Di Candia A, Mancino PV, et al. The Relationships Between Ataxia and Cognition in Spinocerebellar Ataxia Type 2. Cerebellum. 2020 Feb;19(1):40-7.

[16] Giocondo F, Curcio G. Spinocerebellar ataxia: a critical review of cognitive and socio-cognitive deficits. Int J Neurosci. 2018 Feb;128(2):182-91.

[17] Santos de Oliveira LA, Martins CP, Horsczaruk CHR, Lima da Silva DC, Martins JVP, Vasconcelos LFR, et al. Decreasing fall risk in spinocerebellar ataxia. J Phys Ther Sci. 2015 Apr;27(4):1223-5.

[18] Velázquez-Pérez L, Rodríguez-Diaz JC, Rodríguez-Labrada R, Medrano-Montero J, Aguilera Cruz AB, Reynaldo-Cejas L, et al. Neurorehabilitation Improves the Motor Features in Prodromal SCA2: A Randomized, Controlled Trial. Mov Disord. 2019 Jul;34(7):1060-8.

[19] de Oliveira LAS, Martins CP, Horsczaruk CHR, da Silva DCL, Vasconcellos LF, Lopes AJ, et al. Partial Body Weight-Supported Treadmill Training in Spinocerebellar Ataxia. Rehabil Res Pract. 2018;2018:7172686.

[20] Barbuto S, Martelli D, Isirame O, Lee N, Bishop L, Kuo S-H, et al. Phase I Single-Blinded Randomized Controlled Trial Comparing Balance and Aerobic Training in Degenerative Cerebellar Disease. PM R. 2020 May;

[21] Barbuto S, Martelli D, Omofuma IB, Lee N, Kuo S-H, Agrawal S, et al. Phase I randomized single-blinded controlled study investigating the potential benefit of aerobic exercise in degenerative cerebellar disease. Clin Rehabil. 2020 May;34(5):584-94.

[22] Pedroso JL, Braga-Neto P, Escorcio-Bezerra ML, Abrahão A, de Albuquerque MVC, Filho FMR, et al. Non-motor and Extracerebellar Features in Spinocerebellar Ataxia Type 2. Cerebellum. 2017 Feb;16(1):34-9.

[23] Stephen CD, Brizzi KT, Bouffard MA, Gomery P, Sullivan SL, Mello J, et al. The Comprehensive Management of Cerebellar Ataxia in Adults. Curr Treat Options Neurol. 2019 Feb;21(3):9.

[24] Rentiya ZS, Jung BC, Bae J, Liszewski CM, Fishman A, Du AX, et al. Selective Patterns of Cognitive Impairment in Spinocerebellar Ataxia Type 6 and Idiopathic Late-Onset Cerebellar Ataxia. Arch Clin Neuropsychol Off J Natl Acad Neuropsychol. 2018 Jun;33(4):427-36.

[25] Santos LR, Teive HAG, Lopes Neto FDN, Macedo ACB de, Mello NM de, Zonta MB. Quality of life in individuals with spinocerebellar ataxia type 10: a preliminary study. Arq Neuropsiquiatr. 2018 Aug;76(8):527-33.

[26] Abdelgabar AR, Suttrup J, Broersen R, Bhandari R, Picard S, Keysers C, et al. Action perception recruits the cerebellum and is impaired in patients with spinocerebellar ataxia. Brain. 2019 Dec;142(12):3791-805.

[27] Rodríguez-Díaz JC, Velázquez-Pérez L, Rodríguez Labrada R, Aguilera Rodríguez R, Laffita Pérez D, Canales Ochoa N, et al. Neurorehabilitation therapy in spinocerebellar ataxia type 2: A 24-week, rater-blinded, randomized, controlled trial. Mov Disord. 2018 Sep;33(9):1481-7.

[28] Burciu RG, Fritsche N, Granert O, Schmitz L, Spönemann N, Konczak J, et al. Brain changes associated with postural training in patients with cerebellar degeneration: a voxel-based morphometry study. J Neurosci. 2013 Mar;33(10):4594-604.

[29] Aizawa CYP, Pedroso JL, Braga-Neto P, Callegari MR, Barsottini OGP. Patients with autosomal dominant spinocerebellar ataxia have more risk of falls, important balance impairment, and decreased ability to function. Arq Neuropsiquiatr. 2013 Aug;71(8):508-11.

[30] Jacobi H, du Montcel ST, Bauer P, Giunti P, Cook A, Labrum R, et al. Long-term evolution of patient-reported outcome measures in spinocerebellar ataxias. J Neurol. 2018 Sep;265(9):2040-51.

[31] Brusse E, Brusse-Keizer MGJ, Duivenvoorden HJ, van Swieten JC. Fatigue in spinocerebellar ataxia: patient self-assessment of an early and disabling symptom. Neurology. 2011 Mar;76(11):953-9.

[32] Kuo P-H, Gan S-R, Wang J, Lo RY, Figueroa KP, Tomishon D, et al. Dystonia and ataxia progression in spinocerebellar ataxias. Parkinsonism Relat Disord. 2017 Dec;45:75-80.

[33] Coarelli G, Brice A, Durr A. Recent advances in understanding dominant spinocerebellar ataxias from clinical and genetic points of view. F1000Research. 2018;7.

[34] Chirino A, Hernandez-Castillo CR, Galvez V, Contreras A, Diaz R, Beltran-Parrazal L, et al. Motor and cognitive impairments in spinocerebellar ataxia type 7 and its correlations with cortical volumes. Eur J Neurosci. 2018 Nov;48(10):3199-211.

[35] Indelicato E, Fanciulli A, Ndayisaba JP, Nachbauer W, Granata R, Wanschitz J, et al. Autonomic function testing in spinocerebellar ataxia type 2. Clin Auton Res Off J Clin Auton Res Soc. 2018 Jun;28(3):341-6.

[36] Stezin A, Venkatesh SD, Thennarasu K, Purushottam M, Jain S, Yadav R, et al. Non-ataxic manifestations of Spinocerebellar ataxia-2, their determinants and predictors. J Neurol Sci. 2018 Nov;394:14-8.

[37] Isono C, Hirano M, Sakamoto H, Ueno S, Kusunoki S, Nakamura Y. Differences in dysphagia between spinocerebellar ataxia type 3 and type 6. Dysphagia. 2013 Sep;28(3):413-8.

[38] Leonardi L, Aceto MG, Marcotulli C, Arcuria G, Serrao M, Pierelli F, et al. A wearable proprioceptive stabilizer for rehabilitation of limb and gait ataxia in hereditary cerebellar ataxias: a pilot open-labeled study. Neurol Sci Off J Ital Neurol Soc Ital Soc Clin Neurophysiol. 2017 Mar;38(3):459-63.

[39] Ilg W, Timmann D. Gait ataxia--specific cerebellar influences and their rehabilitation. Mov Disord. 2013 Sep;28(11):1566-75.

[40] Chang Y-J, Chou C-C, Huang W-T, Lu C-S, Wong AM, Hsu M-J. Cycling regimen induces spinal circuitry plasticity and improves leg muscle coordination in individuals with spinocerebellar ataxia. Arch Phys Med Rehabil. 2015 Jun;96(6):1006-13.

[41] Fowler EG, Knutson LM, DeMuth SK, Sugi M, Siebert K, Simms V, et al. Pediatric endurance and limb strengthening for children with cerebral palsy (PEDALS)--a randomized controlled trial protocol for a stationary cycling intervention. BMC Pediatr. 2007 Mar;7:14.

[42] Silva RCR, Saute JAM, Silva ACF, Coutinho ACO, Saraiva-Pereira ML, Jardim LB. Occupational therapy in spinocerebellar ataxia type 3: an open-label trial. Brazilian J Med Biol Res = Rev Bras Pesqui medicas e Biol. 2010 Jun;43(6):537-42.

[43] Vogel AP, Folker J, Poole ML. Treatment for speech disorder in Friedreich ataxia and other hereditary ataxia syndromes. Cochrane database Syst Rev. 2014 Oct;(10):CD008953.

[44] Nardone A, Turcato AM, Schieppati M. Effects of balance and gait rehabilitation in cerebellar disease of vascular or degenerative origin. Restor Neurol Neurosci. 2014;32(2):233-45.

[45] Schmitz-Hübsch T, du Montcel ST, Baliko L, Berciano J, Boesch S, Depondt C, et al. Scale for the assessment and rating of ataxia: development of a new clinical scale. Neurology. 2006 Jun;66(11):1717-20.

[46] Jacobi H, Rakowicz M, Rola R, Fancellu R, Mariotti C, Charles P, et al. Inventory of Non-Ataxia Signs (INAS): validation of a new clinical assessment instrument. Cerebellum. 2013 Jun;12(3):418-28.

[47] Berg KO, Wood-Dauphinee SL, Williams JI, Maki B. Measuring balance in the elderly: validation of an instrument. Can J Public Health. 1992;83 Suppl 2:S7-11.

[48] Kusumaningsih W, Triangto K, Salim H. Gait turning patterns in chronic ischemic stroke males and its relationship to recovery: A cross-sectional study. Medicine (Baltimore). 2019 Sep;98(38):e17210.

[49] Faria CD, Teixeira-Salmela LF, Silva EB, Nadeau S. Expanded timed up and go test with subjects with stroke: Reliability and comparisons with matched healthy controls. Arch Phys Med Rehabil [Internet]. 2012;93(6):1034-8. Available from: http://dx.doi.org/10.1016/j.apmr.2011.11.025

[50] Mackintosh S. Functional Independence Measure. Aust J Physiother [Internet]. 2009;55(1):65. Available from: http://linkinghub.elsevier.com/retrieve/pii/S0004951409700662

[51] Linacre JM, Heinemann AW, Wright BD, Granger C V, Hamilton BB. The structure and stability of the Functional Independence Measure. Arch Phys Med Rehabil. 1994 Feb;75(2):127-32.

[52] Ware JEJ. SF-36 health survey update. Spine (Phila Pa 1976). 2000 Dec;25(24):3130-9.

[53] Sánchez-López CR, Perestelo-Pérez L, Escobar A, López-Bastida J, Serrano-Aguilar P. Health-related quality of life in patients with spinocerebellar ataxia. Neurologia. 2017 Apr;32(3):143-51.

[54] Mello NM de, Zonta MB, Teive HAG, Meira AT, Lopes Neto FDN, Silva JT da SN da, et al. Assessment of ventilatory function in patients with spinocerebellar ataxia type 2. Arq Neuropsiquiatr. 2020 Feb;78(2):96-102.

[55] Triangto K, Widjanantie SC, Nusdwinuringtyas N. Biomechanical Impacts of Forward Head Posture on the Respiratory Function. Indones J Phys Med Rehabil. 2019;8(02):50-64.

[56] Zafar H, Albarrati A, Alghadir AH, Iqbal ZA. Effect of Different Head-Neck Postures on the Respiratory Function in Healthy Males. Biomed Res Int. 2018;2018:4518269.

[57] Koseki T, Kakizaki F, Hayashi S, Nishida N, Itoh M. Effect of forward head posture on thoracic shape and respiratory function. J Phys Ther Sci. 2019 Jan;31(1):63-8.

Section 3

Interventions: Medical and Non Medical

Chapter 4

Human Pluripotent Stem Cell-Derived Cerebellar Neurons: From Development to Modeling Cerebellar Ataxias

Roxana Deleanu

Abstract

The most affected cell types in cerebellar ataxias are the cerebellar neurons, which are not readily accessible for cellular and molecular investigation. Pluripotent stem cell (PSC) technology has emerged as an important tool for generating diverse types of neurons, which are used in order to better understand the human nervous system development and pathologies. In this chapter, the strategies for the differentiation of human PSCs toward cerebellar neurons are overviewed, followed by an outlook of their further optimization and diversification by implementing the knowledge from cerebellar development and new cell culture approaches. The optimization stategies are based on the recent progress made in defining the cell populations in mature and developing mouse and human cerebellum. The cellular phenotypes and organization in mouse and human cerebellum are briefly presented, followed by an overview of our current knowledge about their development, which includes pattering, proliferation, neurogenesis, gliogenesis, migration, connectivity and maturation. To date, however, relatively few studies have used induced PSCs (iPSCs) to model cerebellar ataxias and even fewer have looked directly to cerebellar neurons. The reported iPSC-derived *in vitro* models for cerebellar ataxias are reviewed, followed by an outlook of how to improve these models by generating and exporing the cerebellar neurons.

Keywords: cerebellar ataxias, iPSC-derived cellular models, cerebellar neurogenesis, Purkinje cells, cerebellar organoids

1. Introduction

Cerebellar ataxias constitute a very heterogeneous group of diseases in which the motor incoordination is caused by the dysfunction and degeneration of the cerebellar neurons. Although different causative genes or toxins have been identified and several pathological pathways have been investigated, the treatments for these conditions are still largely palliative. Therefore, it is an urgent need for disease-relevant cellular models for studying disease progression and screening for potential therapies.

The rapid development in the field of induced pluripotent stem cell (iPSC) technology offers the opportunity to combine the genetic authenticity of the patient-derived cellular models with the disease-relevant cell types. Human iPSCs have been generated from a wide variety of easily accessible tissues, including skin and blood cells, using methods which nowadays are safer because they avoid the genomic integration of the viral vectors containing reprogramming factors. The potential of iPSCs to differentiate into any cell type of the body was previously explored by the studies with mouse and human embryonic stem cells (ESCs), which are blastocyst-derived pluripotent populations. Both iPSCs and ESCs may offer direct access to study the cells making the nervous system, but straightforth for disease models are the neurons differentiated from iPSCs, generated from patients with a variety of neurologic or neurodegenerative conditions [1, 2].

Although significant advances have been made, most of the protocols for the differentiation of human PSCs into neurons yield cellular populations which can only partially mirror the functional characteristics detected *in vivo*. In addition, most of the available neuronal characterization comes from the studies in rodents and we still know little about the phenotypes that the human neurons have in different stages of their development or degeneration. Nowadays, only few protocols generate efficiently specific neuronal classes, such as the midbrain dopaminergic neurons or the cortical neurons, while for the most neuronal types in the human brain, including the neurons of the cerebellum, the efficiency of the protocols is much lower and additional cell selection methods are required.

As it happened for the generation of other human neural or non-neural cells and especially for the generation of the cerebral cells (reviewed in [3, 4]), the improvements in the generation of cerebellar neurons will definitely come from a better knowledge of the human cerebellum and its developmental pathways.

The human adult cerebellum is the second largest brain part (after the cerebral cortex) and contains around 80 billion neurons (which represents four times more neurons than in the cerebral cortex) [5–8]. These neurons contribute to the complex cerebellar functions, including the control of movements for performing fine-tuning and coordination [9, 10], as well as of cognitive and emotional processes [11, 12]. The morphological and functional organization in the cerebellum, intensively investigated in rodents, is highly conserved across vertebrates [13]. Both human and mouse cerebella contain two lateral hemispheres connected by a region named vermis. The lateral hemispheres are subdivided into lobes and lobules and, together with vermis, covered by a uniformly pliated gray matter forming the cerebellar cortex. Cerebellar neurons have their cell bodies (somas) located in the cerebellar cortex and in the nuclei situated inside the white matter of each cerebellar hemisphere, called deep cerebellar nuclei (DCN). There are four distinctive DCN in mouse (dentate, fastigial, emboliform and globose), while the last two are fused as the interposed nucleus in human [10, 13].

The higher number of lobules in humans makes the cerebellar cortex more expanded relative to mice; in spite of the increase in size, both the volume of the cerebellum as a percentage of the total brain and the ratio of the number of neurons in the cerebellum to the cerebral cortex is remarkably constant across mammalian species, pointing to the concomitant increase of the cerebellum and the cerebral cortex in humans [6, 8, 14–17].

The morphological organization of the adult cerebellum is schematically presented in **Figure 1**. The neurons located in the cerebellar cortex form three laminar structures laying between the internal white matter and the external pia mater: the granular layer (GL, named also the inner GL), the Purkinje layer (PL) and the molecular layer (ML). The GL contains the densely packed granule cells, which are the most abundant cell type in cerebellum and in the whole brain, as well as few other cells, such as Golgi cells (with different subtypes, such as Lugano, globular and candelabrum) and unipolar brush cells. PL is a narrow middle zone

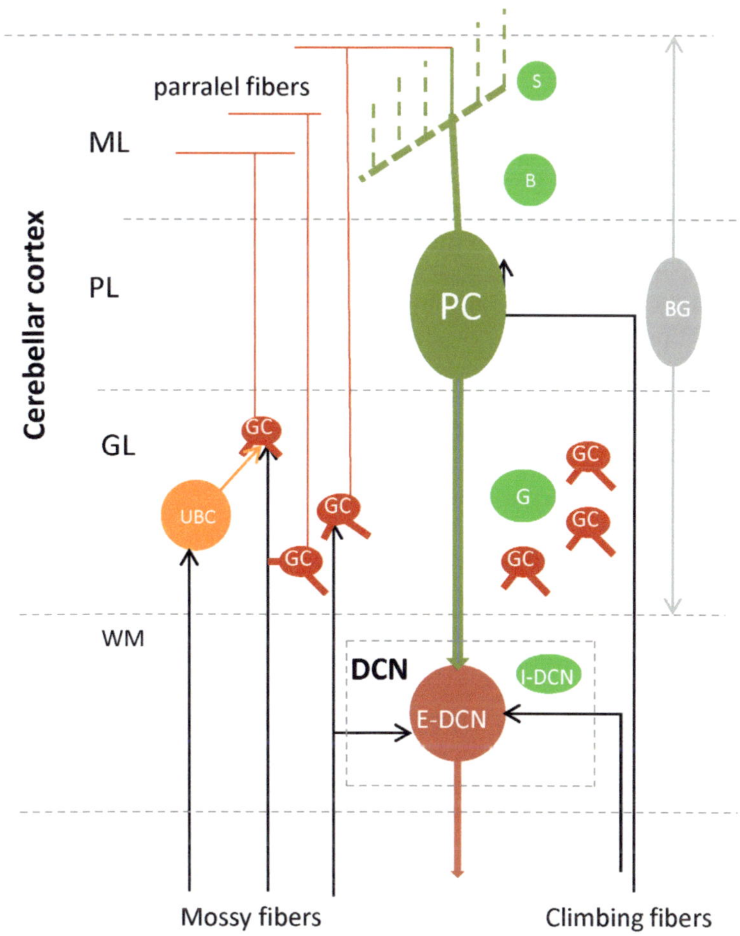

Figure 1.
Cellular composition and organization in the adult cerebellum. The cerebellum contains, from exterior to interior, the cerebellar cortex with 3 layers, the molecular layer (ML), the Purkinje layer (PL) and the granular layer (GL), and the deep cerebellar nuclei (DCN) situated in the white matter (WM). Excitatory (red-orange) and inhibitory (green) neurons are located in the cortex (granule cells (GC), unipolar brush cells (UBC), Purkinje cells (PC), Golgi (G), basket (B) and stellate (S) cells) and in the DCN (E-DCN and I-DCN). GC and UBC receive external afferents via mossy fiber, while E-DCN via both mossy fibers and climbing fibers. PC receive external afferents via climbing fibers and internal afferents via parallel fibers, sending efferents to DCN. BG: Bergmann glia (gray).

that contains the large cell bodies of the Purkinje cells, together with the cell bodies of a special type of glial cells named Bergmann glia. The ML contains mainly cell projections, but also a few entire neurons such as the basket cells located near the PL and stellate cells located near the pia mater.

In addition to the shape and location of their cell bodies, the cerebellar neurons are characterized by other intrinsic properties included in their neurochemical profiles (neurotransmitters, associated neuropeptides and receptors), electrophysiological profiles and, in the recent years, in high-throughput transcriptional fingerprints. Based on the neurotransmitters used for synaptic communication, cerebellar neurons are set into two *main classes*: excitatory neurons, which release glutamate, and inhibitory neurons, which release mainly γ-aminobutyric acid (GABA). Excitatory neurons are situated in the cerebellar cortex (granule and unipolar brush cells) and in the DCN. Inhibitory neurons are localized also in the cerebellar cortex (Purkinje cells, Golgi cells, basket and stellate cells) and in the DCN (**Figure 1**).

Regarding tissue architecture and connectivity, the cerebellar neurons are arranged as repeating units in a highly regular manner, relatively identical in all areas of the cerebellar cortex. Granule cells and excitatory neurons in DCN are projection neurons, while inhibitory neurons in the cortex (Golgi cells, stellate cells and basket cells) and DCN, and the unipolar brush cells are interneurons. Granule cells receive excitatory signals from neurons of the brainstem or spinal cord, mainly with a station in the middle or inferior cerebellar peduncle, *via* the mossy fiber afferents. The information from ~25 million mossy fibers is dispersed to ~50 billion granule cells, but each dendrite apparently synapses with a single mossy fiber, in this way promoting combinatorial encoding and enhanced processing of sensory input to the cerebellum. Unipolar brush cells receive sensorimotor signals *via* mossy fibers, each cell forming a specialized giant synaptic junction with a single mossy fiber terminal. Their axons branch locally within the GL, where an intrinsic system superimposes on the canonical extrinsic mossy fiber system (reviewed in [15]).

The axons of granule cells project to the ML, where they form the parallel fibers, which intercept the dendrites of Purkinje cells at right angles. There are ~200 granule cells per Purkinje cell in mice, while in humans there are 3000 granule cells *per* Purkinje cell [8]. Purkinje cell bodies form a monolayer in the middle of PL, each neuron sending a monoplane-oriented expansive dendritic tree with thousands of little spines into the ML, while its axon projects towards and connects with one neuron in the DCN. In addition to the inputs from granule cells, each Purkinje cell receives excitatory signals from climbing fibers arising from the inferior olive neurons in the medulla (which receives sensory information from the cortex). Purkinje cells convey the results of the analysis of afferent information to the excitatory neurons in DCN, which form the main cerebellar output. Each excitatory neuron in DCN receives inputs from several Purkinje cells, but also inputs from the spinocerebellar tract *via* the mossy fibers and from the inferior olive *via* the climbing fibers. Excitatory neurons in DCN send projections back to the brainstem and to motor cortex *via* the thalamus [18, 19].

Remarkably, Purkinje cells can exhibit two distinct types of action potential, with simple and complex spikes. The simple spikes represent an autonomous pacemaker activity, with very little variability between spiking intervals, firing in absence of synaptic inputs. The simple spikes can be modulated by inputs from mossy fiber *via* the parralel fibers. Inhibitory interneurons in the ML, i.e. the stellate and basket cells, also influence circuit topography by making synapses with the dendritic tree and modulating the activity level of Purkinje cells. Additionally, Purkinje cells can evoke complex climbing fiber inputs. Integration of the inputs from climbing fibers and parralel fibers in Purkinje cells generates a unique form of heterosynaptic plasticity, that has been shown to underlie the motor learning [18, 20, 21]. In line with the recent multimodal characterization of the cerebral cortical neurons [22], a deeper investigation of the electrical profiles in human cerebellum is expected from the new Patch-seq techniques [23, 24].

A more extensive neuronal characterization was recently performed by high throughput sequencing, including single-cell sequencing for mouse and human cerebellar tissue [25, 26]. In spite of their quite regular morphology, the cerebellar neurons in each subclass appear as a heterogeneous population, different subsets being defined by several molecular cues, including co-neurotransmitters (e.g. glycine) and neuromodulators (e.g. calbindin, parvalbumin). Markers of some subclasses are related to the position in the cerebellar areas (reviewed in [27]). In addition, a comparative high throughput analysis of mouse versus human cerebellar cells using single cell-RNA sequencing showed that several genes are expressed in human but not in mouse Purkinje cells and confirmed at protein level the expression of novel and specific human Purkinje cell markers, in line with the data from the cerebral cortex [28, 29].

Recent progress in genetic technologies has significantly clarified how the cerebellar cells and their circuits are formed in model organisms, especially in mouse [30–33]. Remarkable advances were made not only in defining of the molecular phenotypes and the differentiation pathways for most of the neural progenitors, but also in understanding of how these synchronize for forming neuronal circuits. Purkinje cells have major roles also during development [34]. They orchestrate the long lasting neurogenesis of the granule cells, the most abundant local excitatory neurons, and the maturation of the local inhibitory neurons, which reciprocally respond by helping in their own maturation.

The human-specific morphological and functional attributes were intensively studied over the last two decades, including for the development of the cerebellum. Mouse mutants for different genes related to developmental diseases affecting the cerebellum in humans demonstrated a considerable evolutionary conservation of the molecular programs across species, but also revealed some human-specific differences. Recent investigations of the developing human cerebellum have emphasized some differences in the organization of the cerebellar progenitor pools. Other human specific differences have been outlined by the single-cell sequencing of different brain cells, including cells in the cerebellum. These high throughput results point out that we still have much to learn about the human cerebellar development, composition and functions.

To what extent can or could the cellular diversity in the adult human cerebellum, and, in the same time, the spatial precision in its organization *in vivo* be reproduced by the PSC-related differentiation protocols? Which would be a proper human model for cerebellum development and cerebellar diseases?

The reported strategies for the differentiation of human PSCs toward cerebellar neurons, especially toward Purkinje cells, are reviewed in this chaper, followed by an outlook of their further optimization and diversification by implementing the knowledge from cerebellar development and new cell culture approaches. This outlook incudes an overview of the recent progress made in defining the cell populations in developing mouse and human cerebellum, followed by our current knowledge about their development, which includes pattering, proliferation, neurogenesis, gliogenesis, migration, connectivity and maturation. This knowledge is also the basis for the establishment and optimization of the PSC-derived models for cerebellar ataxias. An overview of the reported *in vitro* patient-derived iPSC approaches for modeling cerebellar ataxias is presented, followed by an outlook of some challenges that remains to be overcome.

2. Differentiation of pluripotent stem cells toward cerebellar neurons

Over the past 20 years, human PSCs, including the ESCs and the iPSCs [35–38], have revolutionized the research on human development and diseases, particularly for the nervous system. Considerable progress has been made in converting human PSC into different types of neural progenitors, from which some continued to differentiate toward different classes of neurons, *in vitro* or after xenotransplantation.

Most of the reported human PSC-based protocols are an adaptation of the protocols that were previously developed for mouse ESCs, which reflect, to a various extent, different stages of neural differentiation in mouse embryo. On this line, the differentiation of the human PSCs is expected to reflect different stages of neural differentiation in human embryonic and fetal stages. Remarkably, recent data have demonstrated that several protocols starting from human PSCs produced authentic neurons and structured brain-like tissues, including the cerebral cortex, the most complex structure in the human brain. However, many questions remain about the extent to which the relative simplistic *in vitro* settings could reproduce the high complexity of the adult brain structures, both in cell diversity and connectivity (reviewed in [3, 39]).

For the neurons making the human cerebellum, the progress of *in vitro* differentiation protocols was a lot slower comparing to other neuronal populations, such as the spinal cord motoneurons, midbrain dopaminergic neurons, and glutamatergic and GABAergic cortical neurons, between many others. The main reason is the complexity of the cerebellar development, which was only partially and only recently deciphered (overviewed in the next section), while the developmental mechanisms for the spinal cord, midbrain and cerebral cortex were much faster and deeper investigated [40–43].

Increasing understanding of cerebellar development has allowed the elaboration of several protocols in the last years, which made the production of some classes of cerebellar neurons possible, with increasing efficiencies. These protocols were implemented in 2D and 3D cell cultures, or in their combination. As for other brain regions, the differentiation protocols include "directed" steps, meaning controlled differentiation by using extrinsic manipulation approaches, but also steps in which the differentiation advances spontaneously. Most of the protocols use morphogens/growth factors or small molecules with similar functions, which are sequentially administered to mimic the environment *in vivo*.

Two early studies implemented the mouse ESCs differentiation into cerebellar neurons, using different approaches [44, 45], which were followed by several protocols aimed to increase their efficiency. Su et al. [45] used non-adherent ESC cell clusters in serum-free medium supplemented with fibroblast growth factor 2 (FGF2) and insulin. The cellular spheroids, named serum-free embryoid bodies (SFEB, even though they contained mainly undifferentiated cells in this stage), gradually differentiated into more complex 3D cell aggregates containing a mixture of progenitor cells and neurons, which included some granule cell progenitors and few neurons expressing early Purkinje cell markers. Following the same conditions, Muguruma et al. [46] showed that the FGF2-treated neural progenitors presented a broad fate, but some cells organized in tissue-like structures resembling the cerebellum origin in the embryo. These 3D cell aggregates further formed brain organoids, which contained some areas organized as a primitive cerebellar tissue. When cyclopamine, a sonic hedgehog (SHH) antagonist, was added to block the spontaneous ventralization, the proportion of cerebellar cells was increased, including 35–42% Purkinje cell progenitors by day 11 of ESC differentiation. Additionally, this study introduced the selection of the cerebellar progenitor cells, addressing to a cell-surface marker expressed in this population (Kirrel2/Neph3). The selected cells survived and integrated into the mouse cerebellum following *in utero* transplantation at embryonic day (e) 15.5, but their surviving and differentiation into Purkinje cells *in vitro* was possible only in co-culture with dissociated mouse postnatal cerebellar cells [47]. Following the same protocol, Tao et al. [48] showed that the cerebellar organotypic slices prepared from mice at postnatal day (p) 6–8 supply an appropriate trophic environment for the differentiation and maturation of ESC-derived Purkinje cells. Remarkably, after 28 days in co-culture, they showed the same characteristics as the neonatal Purkinje cells.

Salero and Hatten [44] succeeded in generating mouse ESC-derived granule cells at a relatively high efficiency by implementing a protocol in 2D culture based on step-related treatments with different morphogens. FGF8, WNT1 and retinoic acid (RA) were used in the first step, while bone morphogenic proteins (BMPs) were used in the next step to obtain the granule cell progenitors, which were next proliferated with SHH and Jagged1 and showed markers expressed in GL *in vivo*.

Again, for differentiation and maturation, granule cell progenitors were co-cultured with either postnatal mouse cerebellar neurons or glial-conditioned medium and the resulted neurons resembled the neonatal counterparts.

The pioneering studies of mouse ESC cerebellar differentiation were next translated to human PSCs and subsequently refined (**Table 1**). The protocol of Muguruma et al. [46] in 3D culture was applied to human ESC and iPSCs [49, 50, 52]. Human progenitor cells self-organized in polarized neuroepithelium containing around 10% KIRELL2+ cells after 20 days. Muguruma et al. [50] also refined this protocol and followed a long-term ESC differentiation in 3D culture, an approach which resembled the first generation of human brain organoids. They found that the dorsal hindbrain patterning is more efficient for human cells without cyclopamine. Sequential addition of FGF19 and stromal cell-derived factor 1 (SDF1) generated approximately 28% KIRREL2+ cells (representing the progenitors of the cerebellar inhibitory neurons) and 18% ATOH1+ cells (representing the progenitors of the cerebellar excitatory neurons) by day 35. As for the mouse protocol,

General procedure	Hindbrain patterning	Cerebellar progenitors		Cell selection	Neuronal maturation	References
		VZ	RL			
3D cell cultures • spontaneous IsO induction • cerebellar organoids	FGF2, insulin, cyclopamin	KIRREL2+		—	on organotypic cerebellar slices (rat, human)	Wang [49]
	• FGF2, insulin • FGF19 • SDF1	KIRREL2+	ATOH1+	KIRREL2+ VZ progenitors by FACS	co-culture with postnatal mouse granule cell progenitors <150 days	Muguruma [50], Ishida [51]
	• FGF2, insulin, TGFβ antagonist	KIRREL2+	ATOH1+	—	co-culture with e18.5 mouse cerebellar progenitors <70 days	Watson [52]
2D cell cultures • controlled neural induction (Noggin, SB431542) • directed dorsal hindbrain patterning • selection of neurons	FGF8b and RA	KIRREL2+	ATOH1+	ATOH1-GFP+ by FACS	cell transplantation in mouse brain	Erceg [53]
	D0–4: WNT agonist (CHIR-99021) D4–12: FGF8b	KIRREL2+	—	THY+ immature neurons by MACS	co-culture with mouse granule cells	Sundberg [54]
	D0–4: WNT agonist (CHIR-99021) 1.5 μM D4–12: FGF8b (100 ng/ml) D12–24: BDNF	EN1/2 GBX2 (D6)	—	(D22) Negative selection for GD3 by immunopanning Positive selection for NCAM1+ immature neurons by MACS	co-culture with mouse cerebellar glia < 65 days and next with granule cells < 89 days	Buchholz [28]

Table 1.
Reported protocols for the differentiation of human PSCs toward cerebellar neurons.

KIRREL2+ cells were subsequently selected by fluorescence activated cell sorting (FACS) and differentiated into Purkinje cells in co-culture with murine granule cell progenitors. The *in vitro* differentiation of the KIRREL2+ cells for 10 days generated ~45% Purkinje cell progenitors.

Other approaches aimed to increase the proportion of human ESC-derived cerebellar cells by applying the hindbrain patterning conditions tested for mouse ESCs [44]. Erceg et al. [53, 55] treated human ESCs aggregates with FGF8b and RA, followed by a manual selection of the neuroepithelial cells organized in polarized structures. This procedure yielded, after further differentiation, a heterogeneous population expressing markers of granule cells, Purkinje cells and glial cells. In a more directed differentiation approach, Sundberg et al. [54] used the WNT agonist CHIR99021, FGF8b and FGF2 for pattering the neuroepithelial cells resulted from the parallel neural induction of human ESCs with dual-SMAD inhibition [56]. The patterned progenitors gradually express the hindbrain, cerebellar and Purkinje cell progenitor markers, such as EN1/2, GBX2, PTF1a, KIRREL2 and SKOR2. Between days 24 and 48 of differentiation, markers of GABAergic phenotype and markers of immature Purkinje cells, such as PCP2, were detected. In order to enrich for the Purkinje cell population, instead of the previously used cell sorting for KIRELL2, Sundberg et al. [54] implemented the THY1+ cell selection, a method previously used to purify mouse Purkinje cells from primary cerebellar cultures [57]. The sorted THY1+ cells further matured into Purkinje cells expressing the early Purkinje cells marker PCP2 (or L7). The same team further optimized the directed differentiation protocol [28], by quantifying the effect of patterning molecules on directing the cerebellar cell phenotypes. They found that the combination of the GSK3 inhibitor CHIR99021 (1.5 μM) for 4 days with FGF8b (100 ng/ml) between days 5 and 12 of differentiation generated the highest proportion of Purkinje cell progenitors. From days 12 to 24, neural cell expressing the cerebellar marker KIRREL2 gave rise to increasing numbers of adjacently located cells expressing Purkinje cell markers. As early as day 35 of differentiation, subpopulations of iPSC-derived cells expressed markers of the primary cerebellar progenitor cells. The postmitotic Purkinje cell marker PCP2 was observed starting from day 18 onward. Flow cytometry analysis showed that ~23% of cells expressed PCP2 at day 24 of differentiation. A changing element of this protocol was the selection of the immature human PSC-derived Purkinje cells in two steps, a negative selection by GD3 immunopanning and a positive selection by magnetic cell sorting (MACS) with NCAM antibodies [28].

As for the mouse cerebellar neurons, the conditions used for the *in vitro* maturation of the Purkinje cells and granule cells generated from human PSC were undefined, based on co-culture with different cerebellar tissue-derived populations (**Table 1**). The maturation into functional Purkinje neurons has so far been achieved in undefined conditions by co-culturing with either cerebellar granule cell precursors isolated from murine embryos [50–52], or with fetal or postnatal cerebellar organotypic slices [48, 49]. A protocol adapted from Muguruma et al. [50] eliminated the KIRREL2+ cell sorting and employed the differentiation of human cells in co-culture with e18.5 mouse cerebellar progenitors [52]. Again, markers of the cerebellar proliferative zones were detected at early times of differentiation and around 10% Calbindin+ Purkinje cells were detected from day 50 onward. Following long-term co-culture (up to 150 days), these neurons expressed the Purkinje cell markers L7, Calbindin, Aldolase C and LHX5 [50]. In the study of Sundberg et al. [54], the selected Purkinje cells were co-cultured with mouse cerebellar glia and then with mouse granule cells. With this methodology, human PSC-derived Purkinje cells formed synapses with mouse granule cells and had more differentiated morphologies. However, significant electrophysiological activity, comparable with that of Purkinje cells *in vivo* of the iPSC-derived neurons, was observed only following co-culture with human fetal cerebellar slices [49].

3. Strategies for the optimization of the human PSC-derived cerebellar cultures

Even though the reported protocols have advanced in the generation of cerebellar neuron from human PSCs, they still need a lot of optimization in order to generate homogeneous population of cerebellar neurons in 2D cultures or cerebellar tissue-like aggregated in 3D cultures. Looking at the previous optimizated protocols for generating other neuronal populations, such as the midbrain neurons, the cortical neurons or the cortical organoids, it is relevant to follow again the steps which were gradually applied in order to achieve the efficiency and complexity they offer today (reviewed in [3, 4]). Following this aim, here the development principles of the cerebellar neurons are overviewed, from progenitor specification to neuronal assembles, followed by an outlook of how these principles could be applied for the optimization of the protocols generating cerebellar neurons from human PSCs.

During early embryo development, the human neural tube is formed by the folding of a sheet of neuroepithelium and is progressively closed and regionalized under the control of temporally and spatially coordinated gradients of morphogens secreted by organizer centers. At the end of the neurula stage, corresponding to embryonic day (E) 28, the neural tube is entirely closed and contains, from anterior to posterior, the three primary brain vesicles (forebrain, midbrain and hindbrain) and the spinal cord. Soon after the definition of the midbrain-hindbrain boundary (MHB), cerebellum starts to form at the most anterior and dorsal hindbrain territory. In humans, the cerebellar development is highly protracted, extending from E30 to the end of the second postnatal year. In mice, cerebellum almost completes over a period of around one month, starting from embryonic day (e) 9 and including the first three postnatal weeks (reviewed in [15, 58–60] (**Figure 2**). However, as for the whole brain, the mechanisms of cell differentiation and histogenesis in cerebellum are mainly conserved in mammals. While the development of the mouse cerebellum was intensively studied [15, 30, 32–34, 58, 61–65], the embryonic and fetal stages in human cerebellar development were only recently described in details [13, 16, 59, 60]. Notably, as for the other parts of the human brain, the embryonic and fetal stages of development are not available for cellular and functional studies, and their histological and clinical images represent only snapshots in time for one individual. Conversely, developmental time-course experiments in mice can be conducted on multiple mice of identical genotypes. These studies revealed that the ontogenesis of all neurons and glial cells in the nervous system, including the ones in the cerebellum, follows the same steps of (1) patterning and specification of the progenitor cells, (2) neurogenesis/gliogenesis and (3) migration, histogenesis, formation of the neuronal circuits and neuronal maturation (reviewed in [15, 27, 58, 61, 66, 67]). However, in contrast to other CNS areas, including the cerebral cortex, in which gliogenesis follows neurogenesis [68, 69], glia generation in cerebellum parallels or precedes the long-lasting generation of the granule cells and inhibitory neurons [15, 30, 32, 65, 68]. Even though the main developmental programs are conserved from mice to humans, some important specie-specific differences responsible for the expansion of the human cerebellum have been recently identified [59, 60]. In the following brief presentation, the main morphological, cellular and molecular events in mouse are complemented with the available information in human.

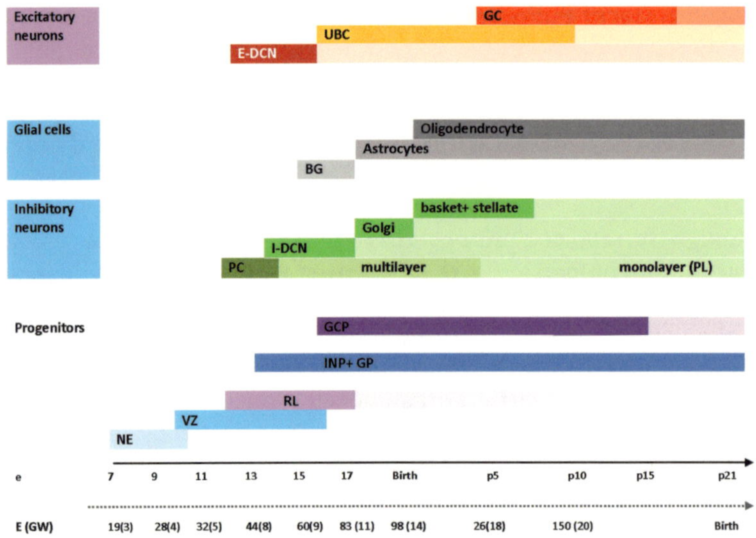

Figure 2.
Timing and the aligned stages in mouse and human cerebellar development. Embryonic days in mouse (e) and human (E). GW-gestational weeks. NE- neuroepithelium (light blue). The cerebellar ventricular zone (VZ) (blue) is the origin of the inhibitory neurons and glial cells. Inhibitory neurons (green) are the Purkinje cells (PC), Golgi, basket and stellate cells, and the inhibitory neurons in the deep cerebellar nuclei (I-DCN). The rhombic lip (RL) (Lila) is the origin of the excitatory neurons in the cortex (Granule cells (GC) and unipolar brush cells (UBC) and in the DCN (E-DCN). Long-lasting progenitor stages for the GC progenitors (GCP-violet), and inhibitory interneuron and glial progenitors (INP and GP, blue). Long-lasting maturation of inhibitory neurons (light green) and of excitatory neurons (light pink-orange), and gliogenesis (gray) stages.

3.1 Patterning and specification of the cerebellar progenitor cells

Several studies in mouse showed that all cerebellar neurons and glial cells originate from the hindbrain region corresponding to the dorsal (or alar) part (or plate) of the first rhombomere (r1) [30, 70]. The anterior limit of the cerebellum is defined by the MHB, named also isthmus, where an organizer center, named the isthmus organizer (IsO), forms early in development and has a major role in the anterior/posterior (A/P) patterning of the midbrain and hindbrain. IsO formation is preceded by a series of pattering events that start in the forming neural plate, where two transcription factors, Otx2 (Orthodenticle Homeobox 2) and Gbx2 (Gastrulation Brain Homeobox 2) define the primitive anterior and posterior domains, respectively [71]. They are further co-expressed in early IsO and then differentially express in the midbrain and hindbrain domains [72]. WNT signaling has a main role in the A/P patterning of the neural tube but also in IsO induction, showed by the loss of IsO in WNT1 homozygous mutants ([73]; reviewed in [74]). Shortly after the primary brain vesicles formation, Fibroblast Growth Factor 8 (FGF8) secreted by IsO patterns the adjacent territories [71, 75–80]. Additional A/P patterning by extra-neurally secreted retinoic acid (RA) defines the metencephalic and myelencephalic secondary hindbrain vesicles. The metencephalon expresses the homeobox gene *Hoxa1*, and formed the first hindbrain rhombomere (r1), where the FGF8 blocks the expression of other *Hox* genes. Next, the selective expression of negative regulators of the activated Ras–ERK pathway in r1 stops the local action of FGF8 [81]. In parallel with the A/P patterning, whole neural tube is patterned also dorsoventrally (D/V). The main ventralizing factor is Sonic Hedgehog (SHH), which by e9 is produced in the floor plate of the metencephalon [15, 74, 82, 83] and secreted into the neural tube's lumen, which at this level becomes the 4th ventricle. Consequently, the alar plate of the r1 territory is patterned into the cerebellar domain (anlagen) (**Figure 3**), while anteriorly situated territory becomes the tectum domain, posteriorly, the r2 domain, and ventrally, the pons domain.

Between e9 and e12.5 and, the cerebellar neuroepithelium undergoes morphological changes: the midline remains as a single cell layer and forms the roof plate, while each lateral part forms two primary proliferative zones, known as the origins of the neural populations in the mouse cerebellum: the cerebellar ventricular zone (VZ) and rhombic lip (RL) (**Figures 2** and **3**) [30]. By e10, the roof plate becomes the second cerebellar organizer center and secretes factors belonging (TGF)-β family, such as the bone morphogenetic proteins (BMPs), the most important dorsalizing factors in the cerebellum, and gradually transforms into the choroid plexus epithelium (ChPe). By e12.5, ChPe additionally produces SHH. Genetic fate mapping proved that the morphogens secreted by IsO, roof plate and floor plate define the cerebellar domains which, in addition to the hindbrain restricted

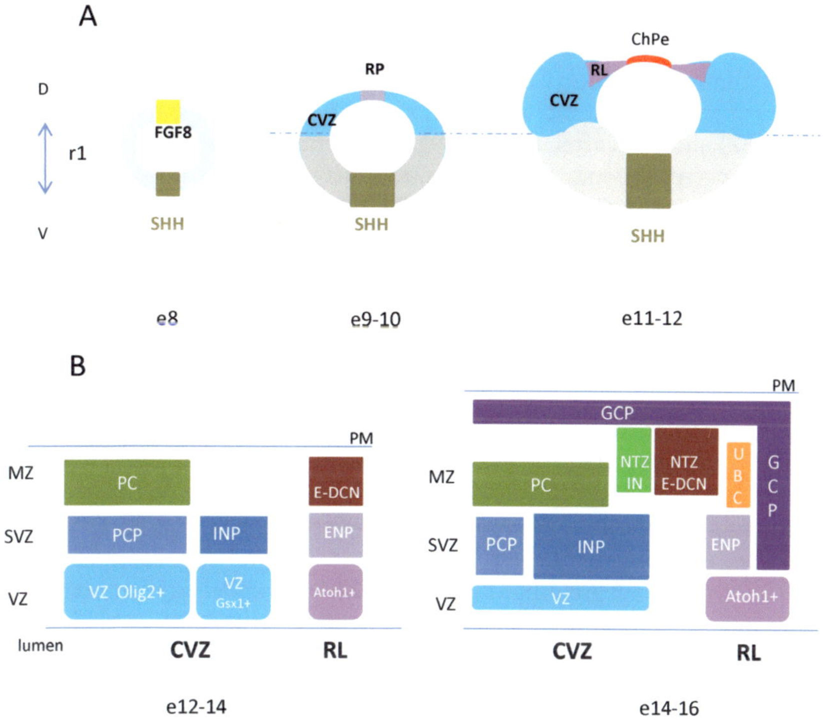

Figure 3.
Stages and distribution of cell populations in mouse early cerebellar development. Formation and differentiation of the cerebellar populations from embryonic day (e) 8 to e16, when all the neuronal populations or their long-lasting progenitors are formed. (A) Between e8 and 12, in the dorsal part of the first rhombomere (r1) of the hindbrain neural tube, the cerebellar ventricular zone (CVZ) (light blue) forms at e9–10, due to the dorsal FGF8 signal and ventral SHH signal, while the rhombic lip (RL) forms at after e10, being visible at the border between the CVZ and the roof plate (RP) (light Lila), due to the BMP signaling from the RP, which forms the choroid plexus epithelium (ChPe) (red). (B) Between e12 and 16, different progenitors arrive in the subventricular zone (SVZ) and mantle zone (MZ) of the neural tube. At e12–14, the Ptf1+ ventricular zone (VZ) of the CVZ primary domain contains the Olig2+ and the Gbx1+ subdomains, which generate the Purkinje cell progenitors (PCP) and the interneuron progenitors (INP, blue) domains, respectively, while the first postmitotic Purkinje cells (PC) already exit the SVZ. The VZ in RL contains Atoh1+ progenitors, which gradually form progenitors of the excitatory neurons in SVZ. They generate first the excitatory neurons for the deep cerebellar nuclei (E-DCN) and at later time points (e14–16), they start to generate the unipolar brush cells (UPC). The RL generates also the progenitors of the granule cells progenitors (GCP-violet), which migrate in waves in the MZ close to the pia mater (PM). In the CVZ, cells representing a subpopulation of the INP domain migrates in the MZ and join the E-DCN in a nuclear transitory zone (NTZ), where they start to differentiate into the inhibitory neurons of the DCN (I-DCN).

expression of Gbx2, show the differential expression of two basic-helix–loop–helix (bHLH) transcription factors: Pancreatic transcription factor 1 (Ptf1) specifies the VZ domain and Atonal homolog 1 (Atoh1, also called Math1), specifies the RL progenitor domain [15, 58, 61, 84, 85].

Each cerebellar progenitor zone forms subdomains with their own spatial and temporal identities, which produce specific neuronal subtypes. VZ-derived progenitors give rise to all GABAergic neurons and glial cells of the cerebellum. VZ-derived neurogenesis starts at e10.5 and continues untill e17 in mouse. Before the neurogenesis starts (~e9), the VZ progenitor domain corresponds to the neuroepithelial cells localized in the VZ of the r1 neural tube (**Figure 3**). Most of the earliest Ptf1a + progenitors upregulate *Kirrel2/Neph3* and oligodendrocyte-specific bHLH gene *Olig2* expression [82, 86], while a small proportion in the early rostral VZ express homeodomain-containing transcription factor gene *Gsx1*. As the neural tube grows, the neuroepithelial cells gradually transform into radial glial progenitors and a subventricular zone appears evident in the VZ domain (SVZvz in **Figure 3**). Ptfa1+ and Olig2+ radial glial cells start to express *Lhx1*, *Lhx5* and *Skor2,* and become Purkinje cell progenitors, located in the SVZvz, which gradually express Neurogenin 1 and 2, start neurogenesis and migrate from the SVZvz. Ptfa1+ and Gbx1+ radial glial cells gradually commit to inhibitory interneuron and glial progenitors. The interneuron progenitors express *Lhx1, Lhx5* and *Pax2*. By e14.5, they become predominant in the SVZvz [87] and soon after start to migrate out of the SVZvz and form transient amplifying progenitor pools. Once all the neurons and transit amplifying progenitors exit the SVZvz, the remaining radial glial cells differentiate into Bergmann glia. The VZ-derived transit amplifying progenitors generate inhibitory interneurons, astrocytes and oligodendrocytes [58].

The neuroepithelium of the RL gives rise to all glutamatergic neurons in the cerebellum (**Figures 2** and **3**), but also to extracerebellar neurons such as the pontine neurons [66, 70]. RL Atoh1+ neuroepithelial cells situated between the roof plate and the VZ domain start their proliferation after the adjacent VZ progenitors (~e10). Also the RL neuroepithelial cells gradually acquire a radial glial phenotype and are patterned in subdomains, which express the paired box gene *Pax6* in combination with the zinc finger genes *Zic* and the homeobox gene *Meis*. First, *Pax6* and *Meis2* expressing progenitors commit to neurogenesis, when they gradually express *Tbr2* and *Tbr1* and generate the glutamatergic neurons in DCN. Later, the remaining RL progenitors co-expressing *Pax6, Meis1, Zic1/2* and *Barhl1* commit to granule cell progenitors, in parallel with the unipolar brush cell progenitors, which upregulate the *Tbr2* expression, downregulate *Pax6* expression and become unipolar brush cells [15, 88].

The cerebellar proliferative zones in human embryos have been only recently investigated. The human cerebellar VZ (gradually forming the SVZ_{vz}) undergoes massive expansion which covers the second month (E30–56), afterwards extinguishing its proliferative potential and remaining as a single cell layer. Conversely, the RL germinal zone remains small during the peak expansion of the VZ progenitors, but starts a significant expansion at around gestational week (GW) 11, when it forms the SVZ_{RL}, which persists long after birth [59, 60].

GABAergic phenotypes. Cerebellar inhibitory neurons, including Purkinje cells and interneurons (Golgi, stellate, basket and inhibitory neurons of the DCN) originate from different subdomains in cerebellar VZ (Ptf1a+), in different waves (**Figures 2** and **3**). Purkinje cell progenitors (expressing Skor2, Lhx1/5 and Corl2) gradually express Neurog1/2 and start neurogenesis, which in mouse is completed at e12.5. Once in the postmitotic stage, Purkinje cells start a short distance radial migration alongside the radial glial processes toward the mantle zone where they stack in a transient multilayered structure named the Purkinje cell plate and gradually express markers such as Purkinje cell protein 2 (Pcp2, named also L7), Pcp4 and Calbindin 1 (Calb1) [15, 64]. In postnatal stages, due to extensive cerebellar expansion, multilayered Purkinje cells gradually form a monolayer while each neuron starts the development of its characteristic extensive and flattened dendritic arbor and the expression of mature markers synaptic markers [30, 58, 89].

In humans, all Purkinje cells are generated before the 8th GW, which places them among the earliest-born central neurons. They start to migrate at E44 outwards from the VZ along radial glial projections to the pial surface. A broad Purkinje cell multilayer extending in the mantle zone is evident between the GW 10 and 13 GW, while a monolayer distribution is achieved by GW 20–24 (**Figure 2**). Human Purkinje cells start to develop their characteristic extensive and flattened dendritic arbors and long axons in the early fetal stages, their final maturation being achieved postnatally, in a 6-fold longer period than in mice [59, 60, 90, 91].

Contrary to the Purkinje cells, which are postmitotic already into the cerebellar SVZvz, the Gbx1+ progenitors expressing the paired homeobox gene *Pax2* migrate in several waves from the SVZvz to the mantle zone, where they start to express the neurogenic genes *Neurog1* or *Ascl1* and differentiate into Pax2+ interneurons. In the first wave (from ~e10.5), the interneuron progenitors migrate to the rostral end of the cerebellar anlage in a Nuclear Transitory Zone (NTZ), which is transient zone for the DCN assembly [15]. After the progenitors settle near the already established excitatory neurons, they produce the inhibitory interneurons of the DCN. In later stages of development, NTZ is gradually organized into distinct DCN. In the second wave (from ~e13.5), the interneuron progenitors migrate to the Purkinje cell multilayer, continue their migration in the developing white matter and postnatally reach the developing granular layer where they generate postmitotic Golgi cells. At later stages, interneuron progenitors migrate radially in the white matter, continue to proliferate in a transit amplifying center and eventually generate the stellate and basket cells in the ML [78, 92]. In parallel with the late interneurons progenitors, the progenitors of astrocytes and oligodendrocytes continue to proliferate in the developing white matter (**Figure 2**).

Glutamatergic cerebellar neurons (excitatory neurons in DCN, granule cells and unipolar brush cells) originate from different subdomains of the RL, in different waves (**Figures 2** and **3**). The first cells leaving from the RL are the newborn excitatory neurons in DCN. Next, the granule cell progenitors migrate in waves out of the RL, where they continue the proliferation. In the first wave (e10.5–12.5), discrete subpopulations of rostrally situated Atoh1+ cells gradually upregulate *Pax6*, *Meis2*, *Lhx9 Tbr2* and *Tbr1* and become newborn glutamatergic neurons, which migrate rostrally and tangentially to the NTZ [15, 88, 93]. The allocation of a temporal framework of different DCN components is accompanied by a characterized sequence of transcriptional maturation that results in the first born neurons for the lateral nucleus (projecting to midbrain and thalamus), followed by neurons for the medial (fastigial) group.

The second wave covers middle to late embryonic stages, when Pax6+ granule cell progenitors leave the RL, migrate out toward the pial surface and undergo a prolonged expansion in a secondary germinal zone, or a second transit amplifying center, named the external granular layer (EGL) [64]. Granule cell progenitors retain the expression of *Atoh1* and migrate into the mantle zone where they express *Tbr2* and continue to proliferate to form the EGL [88]. During the early postnatal period, multiple mitogenic pathways expand the EGL. Peak EGL proliferation occurs around p7 and is complete by p15 (**Figure 2**). The main mitogen is the SHH, secreted by the underlying Purkinje cells [94], but also Jag1, a ligand the Notch2, acts locally in the EGL [95]. Exponential granule cell proliferation in the EGL drives cerebellar growth and foliation [96]. BMP4 and WNT3 secreted by the ChPe promote cell-cycle exit and neurogenesis [15]. The postmitotic granule cells downregulate *Atoh1* and upregulate *NeuroD1* [15]. Newborn granule cells migrate tangentially within the EGL and then exit the EGL migrating radially inwardly along Bergmann glial fibers, trailing a long T-shaped axon behind, interact with the flat, elaborate dendrites of Purkinje cells and form the parallel fibers in ML. Migrating granule cells settle below the developing PL to form the internal granule layer (IGL, corresponding to the adult GL), achieving the final laminar arrangement of the mature cerebellum, from where they extend dendrites to form synapses with mossy fiber afferent axons [15, 58].

Unipolar brush cell differentiation parallels the granule cell progenitor waves (**Figure 2**). Unipolar brush cells are born starting with e13.4, while continuing to p0–1. Progenitors of the unipolar brush cells express Wnt1 early in development (e10.5–13.5), but this expression is downregulated before they migrate from the RL. The newly generated neurons remain in the RL for an additional 1–2 days, after which they exit RL and migrate dorsally through the white matter to their final destination. Most unipolar brush cells reach the IGL by p10, several days before granule cell neurogenesis is complete. Their final maturation occurs between p2 and p28, which seems to coincide with the establishment of the first synaptic contacts with external mossy fibers [15, 27, 88].

3.2 Coordinated formation of the cerebellar circuits

The successful construction of the neuronal circuitry relies on the coordinated generation of functionally opposed neurons. Accordingly, the differentiation programs of cerebellar excitatory and inhibitory neurons are interdependent and defined as the coordinated integration of the VZ and RL-derived lineages in local circuits, in both the cortex and DCN. For the DCN, the cell fate of the excitatory neurons appears determined at the RL, in a temporal pattern, while the interneuron progenitors migrate, differentiate and integrate in the NTZ after receiving local signals from the excitatory neurons.

Purkinje cells have a remarkable capacity to regulate developmental events by sending SHH signals bi-directionally. Starting at e16.5 and continuing throughout adulthood, *SHH* expression in cerebellum is restricted to Purkinje cells and Bergmann glia [97]. Dendritic-derived SHH drives the granule progenitor cell proliferation, while axon-derived SHH disseminates to the neonatal white matter and contributes to the expansion of the VZ-derived progenitors for the late-born interneurons and glial cells during the postnatal period [98]. Additionally, Purkinje cells are critical for the terminal differentiation and morphogenesis of the interneurons in the ML, the basket and stellate cells. On the other side, signaling from differentiating granule cells influences the planarity and the elaborate branching pattern of the Purkinje cell dendritic tree, which occurs from p5 to p15 [99, 100]. Additionally, the dendritic differentiation of the interneurons in ML is sensitive to the granule cell-derived inputs, including BDNF signaling [15].

In the third trimester and postnatally, human cerebellum undergoes its major growth, primarily due to the prolonged expansion of the granule cell progenitors. By 10–11 GW, streams of cells which form the external GL (EGL) were observed along the pial surface connecting to the RL. Due to extensive EGL proliferation, human cerebellum increases 5 fold in size between GW 24–40 [90]. Differentiation and maturation of the human cerebellar neurons progress mainly as in the mouse, but there are some species-specific features. Foliation correlates with EGL proliferation and increases dramatically between GW 20–32, as the cerebellum rapidly increases in size and volume. The formation of the Purkinje cell monolayer coincides with the peak of EGL proliferation [89, 90]. The human cerebellar cortex still has a prominent EGL at birth. EGL gradually decreases in thickness as a result of migration of granule cells into the internal GL. By the end of the second postnatal year, EGL is depleted while the thickness of the molecular layer and the length of the PL increase, concomitant with the increasing cerebellar volume [89, 90]. To date, there are few studies about the development of the human interneurons, both inhibitory and excitatory, which represent a minority comparing to the granule cells, but with a major role in the maturation of Purkinje cells and circuit formation [15, 34, 58, 91, 101].

In addition, the single-cell sequencing techniques have been applied for analyzing different stages of mouse cerebellar development [62, 102]. Carter et al. [62] performed single-cell RNA-sequencing and unbiased classification of around 40 thousand murine cerebellar cells from eight embryonic samples (at e10-e17) and 4 postnatal samples (at p0, p4, p7 and p10). Such approach allows for a more comprehensive detailing of the transcriptional and cellular heterogeneity among lineages of interest and can provide a valuable resource for answering further questions related to cerebellar development and diseases. In a similar study, Peng et al. [102] analyzed around 20 thousand cells from mouse postnatal cerebella and looked in addition to the dynamics of interneuron differentiation but also mitochondrial markers and ataxia risk genes. In a complementary approach, gene expression in the postnatal stages of mouse cerebellar development were analyzed by Buchholtz et al. [28] in Purkinje cell populations selected from mice expressing a *Egfp-Pcp2* reporter gene. Again, the dynamics of different pathways of mitochondrial and autophagy genes correlated with the developmental stages of Purkinje cells, which suggest their implication in several neurodevelopmental diseases.

3.3 From development of the cerebellum to the optimization of the human PSC differentiation protocols

There are several steps to be considered for the cerebellar protocols, which practically cover all the developmental stages: from neural induction and dorsal hindbrain patterning to the patterning and proliferation of the VZ-like and RL-like progenitors, to the neurogenesis of the selected progenitors, and lastly to the maturation of the neurons and the formation of the neuronal circuits. Are the previously used neural induction and early patterning conditions (in both 2D and 3D approaches) optimal for the generation of progenitors similar to the ones in the dorsal r1 in the neurula stage, which represent the origin of the neurons making the cerebellum? Are the previously used conditions optimal for the uniform generation of early VZ and RL progenitors? Which factors and what timing would be necessary for a uniform patterning towards VZ or RL subpopulations? Which conditions would be efficient to produce a uniform neurogenesis from different progenitors? What would the defined conditions for the neuronal maturation be? How can the neuronal maturation be faster? How can other neuronal subtypes, such as the interneurons in the cerebellar cortex and in the DCN, be generated uniformly and efficiently?

Some recent strategies were successful for the optimization of the protocols for the cerebral neurons and cerebral organoids. It remains to be checked whether these strategies can be extrapolated for the cerebellar cultures. Again, the solutions may come from the development principles. The main traiectories that could be followed from the human iPSC to the neuronal cell types contained in the cerebellum are outlooked in **Figure 4** and detailed in the following paragraphs.

Improving neural induction and hindbrain patterning. The first step for all the protocols regarding the neural differentiation of human PSCs implies the removing of the pluripotent cell proliferation factors, such as FGF2 and TGFβ. The additional use of several inhibitors such as BMP/Activin/TGFβ pathway inhibitors, alone (such as Noggin) or in combination (dual-SMAD inhibition by small molecules such as

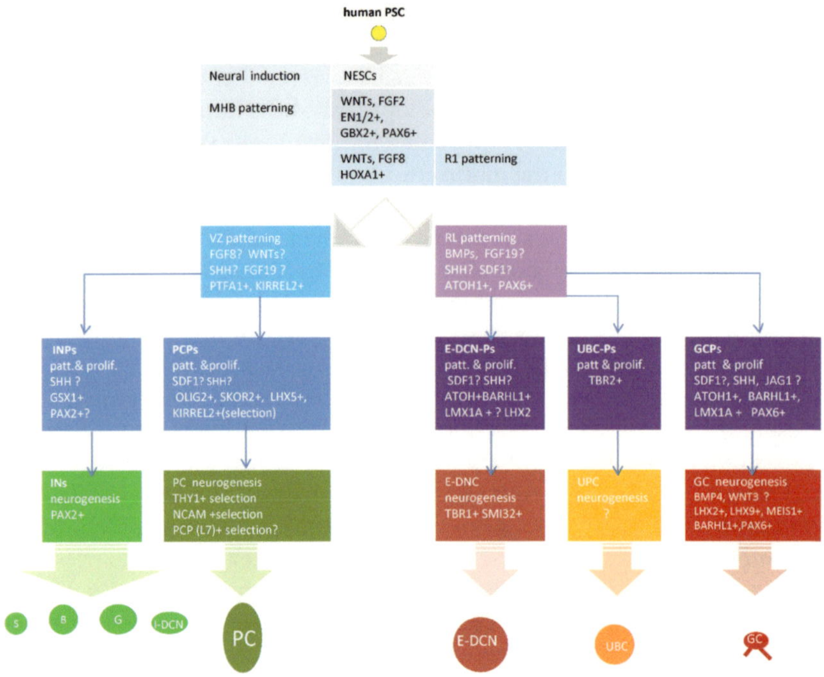

Figure 4.
In vitro trajectories from human induced pluripotent stem cells to cerebellar neurons by combining the differentiation protocols and the developmental principles. The differentiation conditions for some stages (meaning the combination of extrinsic factors, their concentration and time of action in the protocol) are previously established. However, for several steps, it remains to be established which treatments are necessary for patterning and proliferation of progenitor subpopulation in VZ and RL and in the secondary proliferation domains. Some factors which are known to act in the mouse cerebellar development could work also for the patterning and proliferation of human progenitor cells, but many question marks remain. These questions address both the treatments and the specific markers for subpopulation of progenitor cells and neurons.

dorsomorphin or LDN and SB431542) [56], significantly increased the yield of neural induction in human PSCs cultured in serum-free medium, both in 2D and 3D systems [40]. Shortly after neural induction, human PAX6+ neuroepithelial cells acquire a primitive anterior identity, expressing *OTX2*, but no more caudal markers, like *EN1*, *GBX2*, or *HOX* genes [56, 103]. However, this anterior phenotype is transient and, depending on the presence of added or endogenously secreted morphogens such as WNTs, FGFs, and RA, neuroepithelial cells take on a definitive regional identity [41, 104–106].

Some previous protocols used FGF2 for amplifying the neuroepithelial population and showed that, although an anterior phenotype is kept for a few passages in the presence of FGF2, longer exposure gradually patterns human progenitors toward midbrain and hindbrain fates [105, 107, 108]. FGF2 was used by Muguruma et al. [50] for inducing a brought midbrain-hindbrain patterning, including the IsO-like cells, in 3D spontaneously differentiating human PSCs in serum-free medium, for a time approximating the MHB formation in human embryos. However, the reproducibility of this protocol is limited and the efficiency of the neural induction and pattering was not investigated, many cells in the 3D clusters could present a more anterior phenotype (and maybe non-neural phenotypes). Watson et al. [52] proposed the parallel neural induction and hindbrain patterning by using FGF2 in combination with the SMAD inhibitor SB431542 for around 20 days. Even though it showed an increased expression in hindbrain and cerebellar markers, yet the efficiency and the selectivity of this approach was not reported.

The implementation of WNT signaling was shown to increase the midbrain and hindbrain patterning and reduce the spontaneous forebrain patterning in human PSC-derived neural cultures [28, 41, 54, 109, 110]. In Kirkeby et al. [41] and Kirkeby et al. [110], neural induction with dual-SMAD inhibition and pattering were applied in parallel for 9 days. The GSK3 inhibitor CHIR99021 was used at 1–2 μM concentration for patterning the anterior r1 fate. Following this protocol with some modifications, Sundberg et al. [54] applied the neural induction and hindbrain patterning by WNT in the same time, for 12 days, with noggin and 1.7 μM CHIR99021, while in a following study coming from the same group [28], neural induction and patterning with CHIR99021 1.5 μM was applied for only 4 days. In both studies, FGF8b (100 ng/ml) was added from day 4 to day 12 of differentiation, while FGF2 applied at day 10–12 in Sundberg et al. [54] was excluded in the next protocol [28]. However, the resulted cell populations in both studies were not directly phenotyped, but after 16 or 32 days of differentiation, when they contained KIRREL2+ or THY1+ cells, respectively, which were selected by FACS. Further optimization for neural induction and hindbrain patterning requires a deeper investigation, including negative markers for forebrain, midbrain, hindbrain (excepting the r1), and ventral markers (especially for the r1). The dorsal r1 cells should concomitantly and uniformly express GBX2 and EN1/2. Obviously, reporter lines for different genes expressed solely in r1, such as HOXA1, would be very useful tools.

In addition, a study using human hindbrain tissue from embryos at GW 5–7 showed that the hindbrain neuroepithelial cells were stably expandable in FGF2 and EGF conditions, but the short treatment with FGF8 and WNT (for 1 passage) hugely increased the expression of GBX2, EN1 and EN2 [111]. A deeper investigation of the human embryonic dorsal hindbrain tissue could provide hints for the optimization of the human PSC differentiation protocol toward cerebellar cells. The human embryonic hindbrain neuroepithelial cells can be further patterned *in vitro* by BMPs (BMP6, BMP7 and GDF7) and WNT3A to RL progenitors (ATOH1), which generated granule cells after transplantation into the rat cerebellum [111]. Some additional hints are revealed by the pattering of the human embryonic hindbrain tissue. ATOH1 was not expressed if FGF8 was added together with BMPs or if FGF2 and EGF were maintained, FGF signaling appearing to counteract the BMP stimulation [111]. The same factors were applied for the RL patterning from human PSCs (reviewed in [40]). It appears clear that ATOH is not expressed by default, but only after BMP signaling, in spontaneous or directed differentiation approaches. Again, developing human PSC reporter lines for *ATOH* and a deeper phenotypic investigation, including negative markers such the ones express in vicinity of the RL, (e.g. in pons, tectum and neural crest), would be of great help. The same approach is necessary for the optimization of cerebellar VZ progenitors, which are favorized by FGFs and SHH treatments. It remains to be established which treatments with extrinsic factors (combination, concentration and time) are necessary for patterning and proliferation of progenitor subpopulation in VZ and RL, as well as out of them, in the secondary proliferation domain, as long-term proliferative populations (such as granule progenitor cells, interneuron progenitor cells and glial progenitor cells). Some factors known to act in the mouse cerebellar development could work also for human progenitor cells, but many question marks remain. These questions address both the treatments and the specific markers for subpopulation of progenitors and neurons (**Figure 4**).

Increasing maturation of the cerebellar neurons in defined conditions. One of the most consistent observations about human PSC-derived neurons is that they mature relatively slow and often incomplete (reviewed in [3]). An obvious reason is the time in culture: human PSC-derived Purkinje cells are usually kept in culture around

4 months, while they need over 2 years for maturation *in vivo*. An important challenge is the long-term culture and maturation of human PSC-derived cerebellar neurons without the presence of mouse cell/tissue co-cultures. Mature phenotypes of PSC-derived Purkinje cells and granule cells have so far only been demonstrated in co-culture or, more convincingly, by transplantation of differentiated cells into mouse cerebellum. While some of the *in vitro* and transplantation procedures demonstrated the potential of the PSC-derived neurons to mature into functional cerebellar neurons, they also highlighted the need to better understand the factors that promote their maturation. Significant variability in the efficiency to obtain functional Purkinje cells using different feeder cell sources was reported. For instance, feeder-free and co-culturing with rat granular progenitors failed to sustain Purkinje cell maturation and survival, while co-culture with rat cerebellar slices sustained Purkinje cells that nevertheless were devoided of any action potential or spontaneous post-synaptic currents. In contrast, co-culture with human fetal cerebellar slices resulted in electrophysiological active Purkinje cells [49], suggesting that human specific factors, as well as interactions with glial cells [112] are needed for proper maturation. The use of the co-culture system has limitations *per se*, feeder cells introducing inherent variability to the procedure [49]. A growing number of methods for reverse-engineering specific cellular micro-environments and the cells and molecules which constitute these [113] will definitely extend into the cerebellar field. It is likely that the combination of these technologies will help in elucidating key conditions for long-term survival and maturation of PSC-derived cerebellar neurons.

Another approach can come for the optimization of long-term cultures of cerebellar organoid, in line with the extensively investigated field of cerebral organoids [39]. As shown in different previous reports, functional synaptic connections are necessary for maturation and activity of the human PSC-derived neurons, which include glia and target neurons, all of these could be provided in the same cerebellar organoid.

Again, one limitation for most of the human PSC-derived neurons, as for the human neurons in general, is the lack of transcriptomic signatures, to rigorously identify specific types of neurons and to compare their development across species. A recent Metagene projection analysis of global gene expression patterns revealed that differentiating human PSC-derived Purkinje cells share classical and developmental gene expression signatures with developing mouse Purkinje cells. Remarkably, it revealed that the human PSC-derived Purkinje cells matured in co-culture for around two months are closest to late juvenile (p21) mouse Purkinje cells, suggesting that they are relatively mature. Gene expression profiling also identified human-specific genes in human PSC-derived Purkinje cells. Protein expression for one of these human-specific genes CD40LG, a tumor necrosis factor superfamily member, was confirmed in native human cerebellar tissue, arguing for the bona-fide nature of the human PSC-derived cerebellar neurons [28]. Obviously, the routine applications of the single-cell transcriptomics into the optimization steps of the human PSC-derived cerebellar differentiation protocols will hugely contribute to the progress in the field.

4. iPSC-derived models for cerebellar ataxias

The iPSC technology together with the cerebellar differentiation protocols offer the opportunity to indirectly generate and to directly study the most affected cells in patients with cerebellar ataxias, the cerebellar neurons. As schematically presented in **Figure 5**, somatic cells such as skin fibroblasts or white blood cells obtained from patients are reprogrammed into iPSCs, which can be theoretically differentiated into any type of neurons. Ideally, the neuronal differentiation should address the most affected subpopulation in each disease, by following the existing protocols or optimized protocols in the desired direction (using development principles and combining efficient selection methods). Remarkably, for the inherited ataxias, the patient iPSC-derived neurons express the disease mutation in the authentic genetic background and cellular environment, which is not the case in the animal models.

The neuropathological events in hereditary cerebellar ataxias affect both cerebellar and extracerebellar territories. Nevertheless, degeneration and ultimate loss of cerebellar neurons is a neuropathological hallmark in cerebellar ataxias. The affected cerebellar neurons and the responsible genes for several cerebellar ataxias are presented in **Table 2**. Spinocerebellar ataxias (SCAs) are a family of over 40 currently described late-onset dominant diseases, manifesting clinically at middle age and gradually progressing with neurodegeneration in cerebellum and other CNS areas, [136–139] while in other genetic ataxias, such as the autosomal recessive Friedreich ataxia (FRDA) and ataxia-telangiectasia (AT), the disease manifests a lot earlier and, in addition to the nervous system, extraneural territories are affected [137, 138]. FRDA is considered a multi-systemic condition, including central and peripheral neuropathies, diabetes and cardiomyopathy [140, 141].

In cerebellum, SCA1, SCA3 and FRDA involve mainly the DCN, especially the dentate nucleus, but also extracerebellar territories such as the Clarke's column, which present with severe neuronal loss (reviewed in [142]). SCA2 predominantly affects the pontine nuclei, while the Purkinje cells and DCN seem to be secondarily affected. SCA31 is relatively restricted to the Purkinje cells. Although Purkinje cells are predominantly involved in SCA6, degeneration is evident also in the dentate nucleus and granule cells. Therefore, patients with SCA6 show more severe ataxia than those with SCA31. Several SCA subtypes have CAG repeat expansions in the coding region of different genes (http://www.scabase.eu/; [143–146]), resulting in PolyQ elongations in the respective proteins, the elongation size being correlated with the intensity of clinical manifestations. In other SCAs (SCA12, SCA31 and SCA36) or non-SCA monogenic ataxias, such as FRDA, the repeat expansion is intronic, but also in these diseases the cerebellar dysfunction is correlated with the elongation size [147].

Modeling these human genetic disorders in mice has reproduced to a certain extend the neuropathological aspects and has provided some insights into disease mechanisms. Many disease mechanisms that have been explored in mouse models are expected to be recapitulated in patient iPSC-derived neurons. However, some ataxias could not be modeled in mice using the same mutation as in the patients, suggestion that the human-specific environment is essential for the disease to

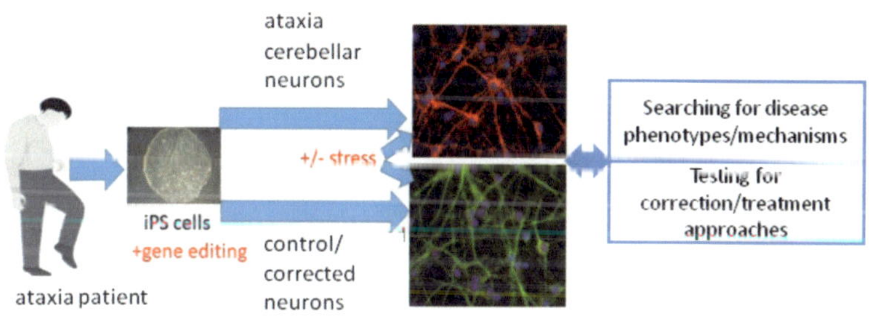

Figure 5.
From ataxia patients to neuronal disease models. Somatic cells from patients with cerebellar ataxias are reprogrammed into induced pluripotent stem (iPS) cells, which can be genetically modified in order to correct the mutation. Patient and control/corrected iPS cells can be differentiated into neurons that are relevant for the cerebellar diseases, such as Purkinje cells. Additional stress or forced aging can be equally applied to the patient and control/corrected neurons or their progenitors, in order to amplify the phenotypic differences resulted from the ataxia's specific mutation.

Ataxia Type	Affected cerebellar neurons	Gene, mutation&location	Affected protein	Human iPSC-derived neurons	Human iPSC-derived models References
SCA1	PCs++, DCN++	*ATXN 1, (CAG)*$_{39–83}$ *exon 8*	Ataxin-1	—	[114, 115]
SCA2	PCs+++, DCN+++	*ATXN2, (CAG)*$_{35–79}$ *exon1*	Ataxin-2	CNS	[116, 117]
SCA3	PCs+, DCN+++	*ATXN3, (CAG)*$_{45–87}$ *exon8*	Ataxin-3	CNS	[117–122]
SCA6	PCs+++, GCs+, DCN++	*CACNA1, (CAG)*$_{20–33}$ *exon 47*	α1A & α1ACT	cerebellar	[51, 107]
SCA7	PCs+++, DCN+++	*ATXN7,(CAG)*$_{38–150}$ *exon3*	Ataxin-7	CNS	[123, 124]
SCA12	PCs+++, DCN+++	*PPP2R2B, (CAG)*$_{55–78}$ *intron*	PP2R2B	—	[125]
SCA17	PCs+++, DCN+++	*TBP, (CAG)*$_{47–63}$ *exon3*	TBP	—	—
SCA31	*PCs+++*	*BEAN1*,(TGGAA)$_n$, (TAGAA)$_n$, (TAAAA)$_n$, or (TAAAATAGAA)$_n$, *intron*	—	—	—
SCA36	PCs+++, DCN+++	*NOP56* (GGCCTG)$_{1500–2000}$ *intron*	—	CNS	[126]
SCA42	PCs+++, DCN+++	*CACNA1G, exon* 5144G > A; R1715H missense	Cav3.1	cerebellar	[127]
FRDA	PCs+, DCN+++	*FXN, (GAA)n, intron 1*	Frataxin	PNS, CNS	[128–134]
A-T	PCs+++, GCs+++	*ATM*, exon, truncating, splicing or missense mutation	ATM	cerebellar	[135]

PCs-Purkinje cells, GCs-granule cells, DCN-deep cerebellar nuclei, +++high ++ medium, +low.

Table 2.
Affected cerebellar neurons and iPSC-derived models for different ataxias.

develop. Additional mechanistic understanding of the network of events produced by the mutation is crucial for the development of effective therapies, as none of the cerebellar ataxias is yet curable, treatable or preventable [143, 145, 147–149].

For modeling cerebellar ataxias, the iPSC-based models present three main advantages. First, most of cerebellar ataxias are monogenic diseases. Second, neurons bearing the mutation, which are not directly available from patients, can be generated *in vitro* from the patient iPSCs. Third, the human neurons generated *in vitro* seem to acquire a molecular profile close to the postnatal age in mouse, as in the previously mentioned Metagene analysis of key gene pathways, which showed that the human Purkinje cells generated *in vitro* have the closest molecular expression with the Purkinje cells in p21 mouse cerebellum [28]. As for many mouse models for cerebellar ataxias a disease phenotype was found close to this age, the *in vitro* generated human neurons are expected to behave similarly and to reveal the disease phenotype in early stage of maturation.

However, as presented in **Table 2**, relatively few studies have succeeded in generating iPSC-based models for cerebellar ataxias. An additional important question for the iPSC-based models is to what extend the mutated gene is expressed in the neurons generated *in vitro*. The most vulnerable and affected cells are neuronal subpopulations, most of them being located in cerebellum. From the reported iPSC-derived models, only a very few implemented the cerebellar differentiation protocols, including the pathways for generating the specific cerebellar cells affected in disease.

A handful of studies published to date addressed iPSC models of PolyQ SCAs (such as SCA1, 2, 3, 6, 7 and 12), non-PolyQ SCAs (such as SCA36 and 42), and other ataxias (such as FRDA and A-T). Most of the iPSC-based models used a generic differentiation towards the neural lineage, as opposed to the generation of specific neuronal subtypes, and very few characterized the neuronal phenotypes. The only reported iPSC-derived models addressing the cerebellar neurons were for SCA6 [51], SCA42 [127] and A-T [135].

For SCA1 and SCA12, only the generation of patient-derived iPSCs were until now reported [114, 115, 119, 125]. Several other SCA models have already addressed the neural phenotypes. SCA2 was modeled by Xia et al. [116] and by Chuang et al. [117] using patient iPSC-derived neural progenitors and central neurons. No cerebellar protocol has yet addressed SCA2, in which both Purkinje cells PCs and DCN neurons are affected. Whereas patient and control fibroblasts showed comparable levels of expression of the disease-causing protein Ataxin-2, its expression was decreased in patient iPSC-derived neural stem cells, which survived shorter in cell culture. Chuang et al. [117] reported that SCA2 neurons exhibited a glutamate-dependent disease phenotype, which are suppressed by anti-glutamate drugs and a calcium stabilizer treatment.

One of the first studies using the generation of neurons from patient iPSCs addressed to SCA3, also called Machado-Joseph disease (MJD) [118]. In this model, neuronal excitation by glutamate promoted an increase in intracellular calcium concentration and proteolysis of Ataxin-3, triggering its aggregation—a hallmark of the disease in patients. This intraneuronal aggregation, (which was also found to depend on sodium and potassium channel function, as well as on ionotropic and voltage-gated calcium channel function), was abolished by calpain inhibition, pointing to a key role of this protease in Ataxin-3 cleavage. Furthermore, intracellular aggregations were not observed in patient iPSCs, fibroblasts or iPSC-derived glial cells, providing a clue for the neuron-specific phenotype observed in SCA3 patients. Hansen et al. [120] differentiated the SCA3 patient-derived iPSCs further into hindbrain neurons that expressed *GBX2* and *HOXA2*. They reported that glutamate loading or calcium increase by ionomycin did not induce Ataxin-3 accumulation in these hindbrain neurons. It remains to be investigated whether this discrepancy comes from a difference in cell types or in the applied protocols. In another study [121], SCA3 iPSCs differentiated into NeuN-positive (postmitotic) neurons showed accumulation of Ataxin-3 in the absence of stress. The activation of autophagy by rapamycin was effective for degradation of Ataxin-3, suggesting that autophagy could be a key for development of therapeutic treatments. Chuang et al. [117] reported that SCA3 iPSC-derived neurons again showed glutamate-dependent phenotypes, which were suppressed by anti-glutamate drugs. Ouyang et al. [122] applied gene editing techniques for the deletion of the expanded CAG in the *ATXN3* gene in SCA3 patient-derived iPSCs, which were further characterized. Such corrected iPSCs will be useful for SCA3 isogenic models. However, no further studies have addressed SCA3 iPSC-derived cerebellar neurons and a directed protocol for the DCN neurons, the most affected in SCA3, is not yet available.

SCA6 is a very interesting case, first, by being one of the three diseases in which patient iPSC-derived cerebellar neurons were generated to date, and second, because of the bicistronic nature of the affected gene, *CACNA1A*. It encodes the α1A subunit of P/Q-type voltage-dependent calcium channel Cav2.1, and the α1ACT, with an identical sequence with the PolyQ bearing C-terminal segment of the longest isoform of α1A [150]. In addition, the gene is expressed mainly in neurons, contrary to the other ataxia-related genes, that are ubiquitous expressed. Utilizing the differentiation method for the cerebellar neurons [50], Ishida et al. [51] differentiated Purkinje cells from iPSCs derived from hetero- and homozygous SCA6 patients [51]. They found that SCA6-derived Purkinje cells exhibit decreased expression of α1ACT and its target molecules, TAF1 and BTG1. They further constructed a disease model in which SCA6 patient-derived Purkinje cells specifically degenerate by depletion of the thyroid hormone triiodothyronine (T3), which is necessary in late stages of maturation. Bavassano et al. [107] differentiated SCA6 patient-derived iPSCs into neurons expressing Cav2.1 and α1ACT, using the same differentiation and stress model as for the SCA3 [118]. The glutamate loading decreased the viability of SCA6 neurons, pointing toward a common pathway of stress response in PolyQ SCAs. In addition, SCA6 neurons showed differences in the expression of several genes previously reported to depend on the transcriptional regulation by the α1ACT, and showed no differences in the electric response of the Cav2.1 channel. Recent high-throughput investigations in the mouse and human cerebellum revealed complex functions of α1ACT [26] and further studies are expected to clarify the role of the mutated α1ACT in cerebellar neurons, especially in Purkinje cells.

For SCA7, in which cerebellar and retinal cells are degenerated [151], Luo et al. [123] reported the generation of iPSCs and neurons from a SCA7 patient, but did not characterize the neuronal phenotype and the disease phenotype. Ward et al. [124] generated SCA7 patient-derived iPSCs and their isogenic lines transduced with either normal or expanded ATXN7. They reported that SCA7 iPSC-derived neural progenitors exhibit altered metabolism and mitochondrial dysfunction.

SCA36 and SCA42 are non PolyQ autosomal dominant diseases, affecting the cerebellar neurons and other neurons. Matsuzono et al. [126] generated motor neurons from the patient-derived iPSCs and recapitulated an increase in RNA foci-positive cells that can be markedly suppressed by treatment of antisense oligonucleotide. SCA42 is caused by a mutation in *CACNA1G*, which encodes T-type voltage-dependent calcium channel Cav3.1 [127]. In addition to identifying the affected gene, [127] reported a model disease for which patient-derived iPSCs were differentiated into Purkinje cells. The SCA42-derived Purkinje cells would provide a useful tool for further phenotype analysis of the mutated CAV3.1, for which the investigation was till now limited to the HEK293 cell line.

For the FRDA, a pioneering work revealed that abnormal expansion of GAA repeats led to upregulation of the DNA mismatch repair protein MSH2 in FRDA patient-derived iPSCs [130]. They reported that the functional inhibition of *MSH2* by shRNA suppresses the repeat expansion. They further reported an inhibitor of histone deacetylase HDACi 109 increased the expression of *FXN* gene and Frataxin protein, pointing to the involvement of histone H3 lysine 9 in *FXN* expression. Polak et al. [131] also focused on epigenetic modifications in FRDA-derived iPSCs and performed drug evaluations. They found that an inhibitor of lysine-specific demethylation enzyme 1 (called Parnate or Tranylcypromine), and the HDAC inhibitor sodium butyrate have transient effects on decreasing the repeats and increasing *FXN* gene expression. Bird et al. [132] also reported a decrease in Frataxin expression in neurons differentiated from FRDA iPSCs, but could not detect abnormality in mitochondrial functions. Hick et al. [133] reported decreased expression of *FXN* and Frataxin, a decrease in mitochondrial membrane potential and degeneration of mitochondria in FRDA IPSC-derived neurons. Eigentler et al. [128] showed a cell-specific decrease of frataxin in disease-vulnerable FRDA iPSC-derived peripheral neurons. Lai et al. [129] and Mazzara et al. [134] generated FRDA isogenic lines. Mazzara et al. [134] demonstrated that the entire intron 1 removal, and not solely the elongation, was necessary for the recovery of the *FXN* expression level in peripheral sensory neurons. Although several studies have provided insights into the pathogenesis of FRDA in cardiomyocytes and peripheral neurons, additional work is required to elucidate the role of Frataxin in other affected cell types, such as the neurons of the DCN.

For the A-T is caused by several mutations in the *ATM* gene [152], Nayler et al. [135] differentiated A-T patient-derived iPSCs into cerebellar neurons and performed RNA sequencing analysis with them. Remarkably, they found that the generated neurons acquired properties of the cerebellum at GW 22 and exhibited disrupted gene regulatory networks related to synaptic vesicle dynamics and oxidative stress.

5. Strategies for optimizing the neuronal models of cerebellar ataxias

Of particular interest in future research in the cerebellar ataxias is the comparison between affected and unaffected neuronal types, in order to identify particular characteristics that render specific neuronal populations vulnerable to a genetic insult which is ubiquitously presented. One of the most crucial needs is to establish a reliable and consistent disease phenotype in a relevant cell population, and those cell types to be generated in relatively large quantities *in vitro* [153].

Differentiation into specific and mature neurons that are the disease targets, such as Purkinje cells for several SCAs, or solely DCN neurons for some ataxias, or both of them for the most of SCAs (**Table 2**), will enable the construction of more reliable disease models [154]. However, the suitability of iPSC-derived neurons for modeling late-onset conditions remains controversial, particularly given the immature, fetal-like phenotypes of the neurons generated from these cells.

Remarkably, in contrast to the immature morphology observed for human PSC-derived Purkinje cells, a recent bioinformatics analysis of their gene expression and developing showed that they most closely resembled late juvenile p21 mouse expression mouse Purkinje cells, when most of the cerebellar disease phenotypes in several animal models start to manifest. This finding suggests that the Purkinje cells are among the most mature human PSC-derived central neurons analyzed to date. This approach also underscores the utility of transcriptomic analysis for analyzing the maturation of human PSC-derived neurons and validates the use of hPSC-neurons for modeling cerebellar ataxias.

Still, it is possible that the disease phenotypes of adult-onset conditions, as the most of genetic SCAs are, may never be fully recapitulated under 2D cell culture conditions, even with directed protocols and optimized maturation. Generation of 3D cerebellar-like tissues as the cerebellar organoids may allow to increasing the neuronal maturation *in vitro*. The next generation or organoids or “assembloids”, which will allow the proper combination of different cell types, including vascularization, can offer a good perspective but also limitations by increased heterogeneity. The multiomics approaches at single-cell level can definitely contribute to understand and quantify this heterogeneity and in the same time decipher the cell-type related disease phenotype.

Another way to model the late-onset diseases is the addition of neural stressors, such as reactive oxygen species, pro-inflammatory factors, and toxins or forced aging, as schematically presented in **Figure 5**. These approaches were already used for modeling several SCAs or other neurologic diseases [153, 155–157]. However, in an ideal situation, these stressors should only exacerbate the disease phenotype, which can be evident in a good model solely by the expression of the mutation in the disease-relevant cells. Another approach is to genetically manipulate the system for forcing the aging, such as by overexpression of progerin in neural progenitors. By this approach, the disease phenotype is expected to manifest *in vitro* in earlier stages of neuronal maturation [155, 156] (reviewed in [158]).

On the other side, recent evidence from cell and animal models indicates that abnormalities in early Purkinje cell development may contribute to the pathogenesis of the ataxias Purkinje cell developmental abnormalities are clearly evident in a wide range of ataxic mouse mutants, including models of the degenerative SCAs [26]. The observed Purkinje cell developmental defects commonly include impaired dendritic arborization, resulting in synaptic deficits affecting CF and PF connections and ultimately altering Purkinje cell physiology. Similar impairments in Purkinje cell dendritogenesis and synapse formation have been described in mouse models of SCA5, and in cell and mouse models of SCA14, SCA1, SCA3 and SCA5. Given the increasing evidence for Purkinje cell developmental abnormalities in cerebellar ataxias, it seems likely that iPSC-derived models, which are capable of recapitulating early developmental events *in vitro*, will be invaluable in unraveling the pathogenic complexities of these conditions. It will be important to better understand the underlying—likely common—molecular mechanisms, by which mutations in distinct genes cause abnormal Purkinje cell development and function [159]. These could offer attractive future therapeutic targets to alleviate motor dysfunction in cerebellar ataxia.

Another limitation in the field of modeling cerebellar ataxias is that most of the studies implemeted the production of iPSCs from a few patients. On one hand, addressing to larger patient cohorts may allow to identifying more accurate phenotypes. On the other hand, for investigating the pathological function of a mutation, the ideal situation is to compare the cells bearing the mutation with control cells with an identical genetic background. The rapid development of CRISPR/Cas9-mediated genome editing is likely to result in significant advances in the field, allowing the correction of disease-causing mutations into iPSCs, which can then be used to create paired isogenic lines to produce better disease models in which far less patient-derived cell lines will be necessary [160]. This was already performed even for the 'difficult to correct' elongations, like in SCA3, SCA7, it is expected in the near future to constitute 'the norm' for all iPSC-derived disease models.

The establishment of efficient, reproducible cellular models of cerebellar dysfunction and degeneration will be important not only in elucidating the molecular basis of these diseases, but also in the development of effective therapies. Establishment of special cell cultures, such as Purkinje cells from patients with cerebellar ataxia, provides opportunities to screen for drugs that may correct the observed disease phenotypes. These cell cultures can be combined with stressors capable of eliciting phenotypes in late-onset conditions and genotypic modifiers of disease progression and drug response. In addition, these cerebellar cell cultures may be used for toxicity screens, to assess the effects of novel compounds on relevant cell types, or for differentiation screens, to identify compounds capable of enhancing self-renewal, maturation or survival of specific cerebellar cells (**Figure 5**).

6. Final remarks

Recent technologies for producing iPSCs from patients combined with the differentiation of PSCs into neural cells and the self-organizing 3D neural tissues have provided a new way to experimentally investigate the developmental and disease mechanisms of the human brain. While several challenges have hindered the generation of cerebellar neurons *in vitro,* starting from human PSCs, some important steps have been made. These protocols, combined with the patient-derived iPSCs, have been further applied for the investigation of several cerebellar diseases. In addition to the "classical" protocols aimed to generate specific types of neurons in two-dimensional (2D) cell cultures, recent progress has been made in culturing cells in three-dimensional (3D) structures, which may better reproduce the tissue organization and complexity *in vivo*, such as the PSC-derived brain organoids. Despite promising results, a number of issues remain to be addressed before the iPSC-based models to be widely adopted. Generation of the disease-relevant cerebellar cells and tissue *in vitro* remains a challenge, requiring a precise understanding of the complex molecular events during the development of each neuronal subtype, and an accurate set of markers by which to identify and characterize the generated cells. The 3D brain models in general and the 3D cerebellar models in particular still wait for improvements, including a better cellular characterization and an increased reliability, in order to contribute to better disease models.

However, human PSC-based models offer distinct advantages for the study of cerebellar ataxias. Cerebellar neuronal models are likely to provide valuable insights into the selective vulnerability of distinct neuronal subtypes, particularly the Purkinje cells. More directed and/or complex approaches will allow for the generation of accurate, disease-relevant models for the study of the molecular mechanisms underlying cerebellar ataxias, and the development of the long-awaited therapies.

Acknowledgements

This work was supported by Austrian Science Fund (FWF), Project P26886-B19, Austria.

Author details

Roxana Deleanu
Institute for Neuroscience, Medical University of Innsbruck, Innsbruck, Austria

*Address all correspondence to: irina-roxana.deleanu@i-med.ac.at

References

[1] Nat, R. and Eigentler, A., (2017). Cell Culture, iPS Cells and Neurodegenerative Diseases" Chapter 13 in the BOOK: *Neurodegenerative Diseases*. Unifying Principles, edited by J Cummings and J Pillai, Oxford University Press, p. 230-241, ISBN 9780190233563

[2] Nat, R. et al., (2013). Human pluripotent stem cells modelling neurodegenerative diseases. In: *Pluripotent Stem Cells* / Book 2, Bhartiya D, Lenka N (Eds.), ISBN: 978-953-51-1192-4 InTech, pp. 447-516

[3] Mostajo-Radji MA, Schmitz MT, Montoya ST, Pollen AA. Reverse engineering human brain evolution using organoid models. Brain Res. 2020 Feb 15;1729:146582. doi: 10.1016/j.brainres.2019.146582. Epub 2019 Dec 3. PMID: 31809699; PMCID: PMC7058376.

[4] Tian A, Muffat J, Li Y. Studying Human Neurodevelopment and Diseases Using 3D Brain Organoids. J Neurosci. 2020 Feb 5;40(6): 1186-1193. doi: 10.1523/ JNEUROSCI.0519-19.2019. PMID: 32024767; PMCID: PMC7002141.

[5] Prestori F, Mapelli L, D'Angelo E. Diverse Neuron Properties and Complex Network Dynamics in the Cerebellar Cortical Inhibitory Circuit. Front Mol Neurosci. 2019 Nov 7;12:267. doi: 10.3389/fnmol.2019.00267. PMID: 31787879; PMCID: PMC6854908.

[6] Azevedo FA, Carvalho LR, Grinberg LT, Farfel JM, Ferretti RE, Leite RE, Jacob Filho W, Lent R, Herculano-Houzel S. Equal numbers of neuronal and nonneuronal cells make the human brain an isometrically scaled-up primate brain. J Comp Neurol. 2009 Apr 10;513(5):532-541. doi: 10.1002/cne.21974. PMID: 19226510.

[7] Herculano-Houzel S. The human brain in numbers: a linearly scaled-up primate brain. Front Hum Neurosci. 2009 Nov 9;3:31. doi: 10.3389/ neuro.09.031.2009. PMID: 19915731; PMCID: PMC2776484.

[8] Lange W. Cell number and cell density in the cerebellar cortex of man and some other mammals. Cell Tissue Res. 1975;157(1):115-124. doi: 10.1007/ BF00223234. PMID: 804353.

[9] Chopra R, Shakkottai VG. Translating cerebellar Purkinje neuron physiology to progress in dominantly inherited ataxia. Future Neurol. 2014 Mar 1;9(2):187-196. doi: 10.2217/ fnl.14.6. PMID: 25221437; PMCID: PMC4159172.

[10] Yamada M. Neuropathology of ataxias. In: Manto M, Schmahmann JD, Rossi F, Gruol DL, Koibuchi N, eds. Handbook of the cerebellum and cerebellar disorders. The Netherlands: Springer, 2013:2327-2347.

[11] Schmahmann JD. The cerebellum and cognition. Neurosci Lett. 2019 Jan 1;688:62-75. doi: 10.1016/j. neulet.2018.07.005. Epub 2018 Jul 8. PMID: 29997061.

[12] Carta I, Chen CH, Schott AL, Dorizan S, Khodakhah K. Cerebellar modulation of the reward circuitry and social behavior. Science. 2019 Jan 18;363(6424):eaav0581. doi: 10.1126/ science.aav0581. PMID: 30655412; PMCID: PMC6711161.

[13] Larsell O. The development of the cerebellum in man in relation to its comparative anatomy. J Comp Neurol. 1947 Oct;87(2):85-129. doi: 10.1002/ cne.900870203. PMID: 20267600.

[14] Herculano-Houzel S. Coordinated scaling of cortical and cerebellar numbers of neurons. Front Neuroanat.

2010 Mar 10;4:12. doi: 10.3389/fnana.2010.00012. PMID: 20300467; PMCID: PMC2839851

[15] Leto K, Arancillo M, Becker EB, Buffo A, Chiang C, Ding B, Dobyns WB, Dusart I, Haldipur P, Hatten ME, Hoshino M, Joyner AL, Kano M, Kilpatrick DL, Koibuchi N, Marino S, MartinezS,MillenKJ,MillnerTO,MiyataT, Parmigiani E, Schilling K, Sekerková G, Sillitoe RV, Sotelo C, Uesaka N, Wefers A, Wingate RJ, Hawkes R. Consensus Paper: Cerebellar Development. Cerebellum. 2016 Dec;15(6):789-828. doi: 10.1007/s12311-015-0724-2. PMID: 26439486; PMCID: PMC4846577.

[16] Keefe MG, Nowakowski TJ. Evolutionary Expansion of Human Cerebellar Germinal Zones. Trends Neurosci. 2020 Feb;43(2):75-77. doi: 10.1016/j.tins.2019.12.005. Epub 2020 Jan 15. PMID: 31954525.

[17] Van Essen DC. Surface-based atlases of cerebellar cortex in the human, macaque, and mouse. Ann N Y Acad Sci. 2002 Dec;978:468-479. doi: 10.1111/j.1749-6632.2002.tb07588.x. PMID: 12582074.

[18] Huang M, Verbeek DS. Why do so many genetic insults lead to Purkinje Cell degeneration and spinocerebellar ataxia? Neurosci Lett. 2019 Jan 1;688:49-57. doi: 10.1016/j.neulet.2018.02.004. Epub 2018 Feb 5. PMID: 29421540.

[19] Jörntell H. Cerebellar physiology: links between microcircuitry properties and sensorimotor functions. J Physiol. 2017 Jan 1;595(1):11-27. doi: 10.1113/JP272769. Epub 2016 Aug 31. PMID: 27388692; PMCID: PMC5199730.

[20] Paulson HL, Shakkottai VG, Clark HB, Orr HT. Polyglutamine spinocerebellar ataxias - from genes to potential treatments. Nat Rev Neurosci. 2017 Oct;18(10):613-626. doi: 10.1038/nrn.2017.92. Epub 2017 Aug 17. PMID: 28855740; PMCID: PMC6420820.

[21] Ramirez JE, Stell BM. Calcium Imaging Reveals Coordinated Simple Spike Pauses in Populations of Cerebellar Purkinje Cells. Cell Rep. 2016 Dec 20;17(12):3125-3132. doi: 10.1016/j.celrep.2016.11.075. PMID: 28009283.

[22] Amiri A, Coppola G, Scuderi S, Wu F, Roychowdhury T, Liu F, Pochareddy S, Shin Y, Safi A, Song L, Zhu Y, Sousa AMM; PsychENCODE Consortium, Gerstein M, Crawford GE, Sestan N, Abyzov A, Vaccarino FM. Transcriptome and epigenome landscape of human cortical development modeled in organoids. Science. 2018 Dec 14;362(6420):eaat6720. doi: 10.1126/science.aat6720. PMID: 30545853; PMCID: PMC6426303.

[23] Mihaljević B, Benavides-Piccione R, Bielza C, Larrañaga P, DeFelipe J. Classification of GABAergic interneurons by leading neuroscientists. Sci Data. 2019 Oct 22;6(1):221. doi: 10.1038/s41597-019-0246-8. PMID: 31641131; PMCID: PMC6805952.

[24] Tremblay R, Lee S, Rudy B. GABAergic Interneurons in the Neocortex: From Cellular Properties to Circuits. Neuron. 2016 Jul 20;91(2):260-92. doi: 10.1016/j.neuron.2016.06.033. PMID: 27477017; PMCID: PMC4980915.

[25] Hodge RD, Bakken TE, Miller JA, Smith KA, Barkan ER, Graybuck LT, Close JL, Long B, Johansen N, Penn O, Yao Z, Eggermont J, Höllt T, Levi BP, Shehata SI, Aevermann B, Beller A, Bertagnolli D, Brouner K, Casper T, Cobbs C, Dalley R, Dee N, Ding SL, Ellenbogen RG, Fong O, Garren E, Goldy J, Gwinn RP, Hirschstein D, Keene CD, Keshk M, Ko AL, Lathia K, Mahfouz A, Maltzer Z, McGraw M, Nguyen TN, Nyhus J, Ojemann JG, Oldre A, Parry S, Reynolds S, Rimorin C, Shapovalova NV, Somasundaram S, Szafer A, Thomsen ER, Tieu M, Quon G, Scheuermann RH, Yuste R,

Sunkin SM, Lelieveldt B, Feng D, Ng L, Bernard A, Hawrylycz M, Phillips JW, Tasic B, Zeng H, Jones AR, Koch C, Lein ES. Conserved cell types with divergent features in human versus mouse cortex. Nature. 2019 Sep;573(7772):61-68. doi: 10.1038/s41586-019-1506-7. Epub 2019 Aug 21. PMID: 31435019; PMCID: PMC6919571.

[26] Du X, Wei C, Hejazi Pastor DP, Rao ER, Li Y, Grasselli G, Godfrey J, Palmenberg AC, Andrade J, Hansel C, Gomez CM. α1ACT Is Essential for Survival and Early Cerebellar Programming in a Critical Neonatal Window. Neuron. 2019 May 22;102(4):770-785.e7. doi: 10.1016/j.neuron.2019.02.036. Epub 2019 Mar 25. PMID: 30922876; PMCID: PMC6533132.

[27] Beckinghausen J, Sillitoe RV. Insights into cerebellar development and connectivity. Neurosci Lett. 2019 Jan 1;688:2-13. doi: 10.1016/j.neulet.2018.05.013. Epub 2018 May 7. PMID: 29746896; PMCID: PMC6222004.

[28] Buchholz DE, Carroll TS, Kocabas A, Zhu X, Behesti H, Faust PL, Stalbow L, Fang Y, Hatten ME. Novel genetic features of human and mouse Purkinje cell differentiation defined by comparative transcriptomics. Proc Natl Acad Sci U S A. 2020 Jun 30;117(26):15085-15095. doi: 10.1073/pnas.2000102117. Epub 2020 Jun 16. PMID: 32546527; PMCID: PMC7334519.

[29] Florio M, Borrell V, Huttner WB. Human-specific genomic signatures of neocortical expansion. Curr Opin Neurobiol. 2017 Feb;42:33-44. doi: 10.1016/j.conb.2016.11.004. Epub 2016 Nov 29. PMID: 27912138.

[30] Haldipur P, Dang D, Millen KJ. Embryology. Handb Clin Neurol. 2018;154:29-44. doi: 10.1016/B978-0-444-63956-1.00002-3. PMID: 29903446; PMCID: PMC6231496.

[31] Legué E, Riedel E, Joyner AL. Clonal analysis reveals granule cell behaviors and compartmentalization that determine the folded morphology of the cerebellum. Development. 2015 May 1;142(9):1661-71. doi: 10.1242/dev.120287. Epub 2015 Apr 1. PMID: 25834018; PMCID: PMC4419279.

[32] Martinez S, Andreu A, Mecklenburg N, Echevarria D. Cellular and molecular basis of cerebellar development. Front Neuroanat. 2013 Jun 26;7:18. doi: 10.3389/fnana.2013.00018. PMID: 23805080; PMCID: PMC3693072.

[33] Marzban H, Del Bigio MR, Alizadeh J, Ghavami S, Zachariah RM, Rastegar M. Cellular commitment in the developing cerebellum. Front Cell Neurosci. 2015 Jan 12;8:450. doi: 10.3389/fncel.2014.00450. PMID: 25628535; PMCID: PMC4290586.

[34] Fleming J, Chiang C. The Purkinje neuron: A central orchestrator of cerebellar neurogenesis. Neurogenesis (Austin). 2015 Sep 17;2(1):e1025940. doi: 10.1080/23262133.2015.1025940. PMID: 27604220; PMCID: PMC4973588.

[35] Takahashi K, Tanabe K, Ohnuki M, Narita M, Ichisaka T, Tomoda K, Yamanaka S. Induction of pluripotent stem cells from adult human fibroblasts by defined factors. Cell. 2007 Nov 30;131(5):861-872. doi: 10.1016/j.cell.2007.11.019. PMID: 18035408.

[36] Thomson JA, Itskovitz-Eldor J, Shapiro SS, Waknitz MA, Swiergiel JJ, Marshall VS, Jones JM. Embryonic stem cell lines derived from human blastocysts. Science. 1998 Nov 6;282(5391):1145-7. doi: 10.1126/science.282.5391.1145. Erratum in: Science 1998 Dec 4;282(5395):1827. PMID: 9804556.

[37] Yu J, Vodyanik MA, Smuga-Otto K, Antosiewicz-Bourget J, Frane JL,

Tian S, Nie J, Jonsdottir GA, Ruotti V, Stewart R, Slukvin II, Thomson JA. Induced pluripotent stem cell lines derived from human somatic cells. Science. 2007 Dec 21;318(5858):1917-1920. doi: 10.1126/science.1151526. Epub 2007 Nov 20. PMID: 18029452.

[38] Bock C, Kiskinis E, Verstappen G, Gu H, Boulting G, Smith ZD, Ziller M, Croft GF, Amoroso MW, Oakley DH, Gnirke A, Eggan K, Meissner A. Reference Maps of human ES and iPS cell variation enable high-throughput characterization of pluripotent cell lines. Cell. 2011 Feb 4;144(3):439-52. doi: 10.1016/j.cell.2010.12.032. PMID: 21295703; PMCID: PMC3063454.

[39] Pollen AA, Bhaduri A, Andrews MG, Nowakowski TJ, Meyerson OS, Mostajo-Radji MA, Di Lullo E, Alvarado B, Bedolli M, DoughertyML, FiddesIT, KronenbergZN, Shuga J, Leyrat AA, West JA, Bershteyn M, Lowe CB, Pavlovic BJ, Salama SR, Haussler D, Eichler EE, Kriegstein AR. Establishing Cerebral Organoids as Models of Human-Specific Brain Evolution. Cell. 2019 Feb 7;176(4):743-756.e17. doi: 10.1016/j.cell.2019.01.017. PMID: 30735633; PMCID: PMC6544371.

[40] Suzuki IK, Vanderhaeghen P. Is this a brain which I see before me? Modeling human neural development with pluripotent stem cells. Development. 2015 Sep 15;142(18):3138-3150. doi: 10.1242/dev.120568. PMID: 26395142.

[41] Kirkeby A, Grealish S, Wolf DA, Nelander J, Wood J, Lundblad M, Lindvall O, Parmar M. Generation of regionally specified neural progenitors and functional neurons from human embryonic stem cells under defined conditions. Cell Rep. 2012 Jun 28;1(6):703-714. doi: 10.1016/j.celrep.2012.04.009. Epub 2012 May 26. PMID: 22813745.

[42] Wichterle H, Lieberam I, Porter JA, Jessell TM. Directed differentiation of embryonic stem cells into motor neurons. Cell. 2002 Aug 9;110(3):385-397. doi: 10.1016/s0092-8674(02)00835-8. PMID: 12176325.

[43] Xi J, Liu Y, Liu H, Chen H, Emborg ME, Zhang SC. Specification of midbrain dopamine neurons from primate pluripotent stem cells. Stem Cells. 2012 Aug;30(8):1655-63. doi: 10.1002/stem.1152. PMID: 22696177; PMCID: PMC3405174.

[44] Salero E, Hatten ME. Differentiation of ES cells into cerebellar neurons. Proc Natl Acad Sci U S A. 2007 Feb 20;104(8):2997-3002. doi: 10.1073/pnas.0610879104. Epub 2007 Feb 9. PMID: 17293457; PMCID: PMC1796781.

[45] Su HL, Muguruma K, Matsuo-Takasaki M, Kengaku M, Watanabe K, Sasai Y. Generation of cerebellar neuron precursors from embryonic stem cells. Dev Biol. 2006 Feb 15;290(2):287-296. doi: 10.1016/j.ydbio.2005.11.010. Epub 2006 Jan 9. PMID: 16406324.

[46] Muguruma K, Nishiyama A, Ono Y, Miyawaki H, Mizuhara E, Hori S, Kakizuka A, Obata K, Yanagawa Y, Hirano T, Sasai Y. Ontogeny-recapitulating generation and tissue integration of ES cell-derived Purkinje cells. Nat Neurosci. 2010 Oct;13(10):1171-1180. doi: 10.1038/nn.2638. Epub 2010 Sep 12. PMID: 20835252.

[47] Baptista CA, Hatten ME, Blazeski R, Mason CA. Cell-cell interactions influence survival and differentiation of purified Purkinje cells in vitro. Neuron. 1994 Feb;12(2):243-260. doi: 10.1016/0896-6273(94)90268-2. PMID: 8110456.

[48] Tao O, Shimazaki T, Okada Y, Naka H, Kohda K,

Yuzaki M, Mizusawa H, Okano H. Efficient generation of mature cerebellar Purkinje cells from mouse embryonic stem cells. J Neurosci Res. 2010 Feb 1;88(2):234-247. doi: 10.1002/jnr.22208. PMID: 19705453.

[49] Wang S, Wang B, Pan N, Fu L, Wang C, Song G, An J, Liu Z, Zhu W, Guan Y, Xu ZQ, Chan P, Chen Z, Zhang YA. Differentiation of human induced pluripotent stem cells to mature functional Purkinje neurons. Sci Rep. 2015 Mar 18;5:9232. doi: 10.1038/srep09232. PMID: 25782665; PMCID: PMC4363833.

[50] Muguruma K, Nishiyama A, Kawakami H, Hashimoto K, Sasai Y. Self-organization of polarized cerebellar tissue in 3D culture of human pluripotent stem cells. Cell Rep. 2015 Feb 3;10(4):537-550. doi: 10.1016/j.celrep.2014.12.051. Epub 2015 Jan 29. PMID: 25640179.

[51] Ishida Y, Kawakami H, Kitajima H, Nishiyama A, Sasai Y, Inoue H, Muguruma K. Vulnerability of Purkinje Cells Generated from Spinocerebellar Ataxia Type 6 Patient-Derived iPSCs. Cell Rep. 2016 Nov 1;17(6):1482-1490. doi: 10.1016/j.celrep.2016.10.026. Erratum in: Cell Rep. 2017 Jan 24;18(4):1075-1076. PMID: 27806289.

[52] Watson LM, Wong MMK, Vowles J, Cowley SA, Becker EBE. A Simplified Method for Generating Purkinje Cells from Human-Induced Pluripotent Stem Cells. Cerebellum. 2018 Aug;17(4):419-427. doi: 10.1007/s12311-017-0913-2. PMID: 29397531; PMCID: PMC6028833.

[53] Erceg S, Ronaghi M, Zipancic I, Lainez S, Roselló MG, Xiong C, Moreno-Manzano V, Rodríguez-Jiménez FJ, Planells R, Alvarez-Dolado M, Bhattacharya SS, Stojkovic M. Efficient differentiation of human embryonic stem cells into functional cerebellar-like cells. Stem Cells Dev. 2010 Nov;19(11):1745-1756. doi: 10.1089/scd.2009.0498. Epub 2010 Oct 7. PMID: 20521974.

[54] Sundberg M, Tochitsky I, Buchholz DE, Winden K, Kujala V, Kapur K, Cataltepe D, Turner D, Han MJ, Woolf CJ, Hatten ME, Sahin M. Purkinje cells derived from TSC patients display hypoexcitability and synaptic deficits associated with reduced FMRP levels and reversed by rapamycin. Mol Psychiatry. 2018 Nov;23(11):2167-2183. doi: 10.1038/s41380-018-0018-4. Epub 2018 Feb 15. PMID: 29449635; PMCID: PMC6093816.

[55] Erceg S, Lukovic D, Moreno-Manzano V, Stojkovic M, Bhattacharya SS. Derivation of cerebellar neurons from human pluripotent stem cells. Curr Protoc Stem Cell Biol. 2012 Mar;Chapter 1:Unit 1H.5. doi: 10.1002/9780470151808.sc01h05s20. PMID: 22415839.

[56] Chambers SM, Fasano CA, Papapetrou EP, Tomishima M, Sadelain M, Studer L. Highly efficient neural conversion of human ES and iPS cells by dual inhibition of SMAD signaling. Nat Biotechnol. 2009 Mar;27(3):275-80. doi: 10.1038/nbt.1529. Epub 2009 Mar 1. Erratum in: Nat Biotechnol. 2009 May;27(5):485. PMID: 19252484; PMCID: PMC2756723.

[57] Heuer H, Mason CA. Thyroid hormone induces cerebellar Purkinje cell dendritic development via the thyroid hormone receptor alpha1. J Neurosci. 2003 Nov 19;23(33):10604-12. doi: 10.1523/JNEUROSCI.23-33-10604.2003. PMID: 14627645; PMCID: PMC6740935.

[58] Butts T, Green MJ, Wingate RJ. Development of the cerebellum: simple steps to make a 'little brain'. Development. 2014 Nov;141(21):4031-4041. doi: 10.1242/dev.106559. PMID: 25336734.

[59] Haldipur P, Aldinger KA, Bernardo S, Deng M, Timms AE,

Overman LM, Winter C, Lisgo SN, Razavi F, Silvestri E, Manganaro L, Adle-Biassette H, Guimiot F, Russo R, Kidron D, Hof PR, Gerrelli D, Lindsay SJ, Dobyns WB, Glass IA, Alexandre P, Millen KJ. Spatiotemporal expansion of primary progenitor zones in the developing human cerebellum. Science. 2019 Oct 25;366(6464):454-460. doi: 10.1126/science.aax7526. Epub 2019 Oct 17. PMID: 31624095; PMCID: PMC6897295.

[60] Marek S, Siegel JS, Gordon EM, Raut RV, Gratton C, Newbold DJ, Ortega M, Laumann TO, Adeyemo B, Miller DB, Zheng A, Lopez KC, Berg JJ, Coalson RS, Nguyen AL, Dierker D, Van AN, Hoyt CR, McDermott KB, Norris SA, Shimony JS, Snyder AZ, Nelson SM, Barch DM, Schlaggar BL, Raichle ME, Petersen SE, Greene DJ, Dosenbach NUF. Spatial and Temporal Organization of the Individual Human Cerebellum. Neuron. 2018 Nov 21;100(4):977-993.e7. doi: 10.1016/j.neuron.2018.10.010. Epub 2018 Oct 25. PMID: 30473014; PMCID: PMC6351081.

[61] Wizeman JW, Guo Q, Wilion EM, Li JY. Specification of diverse cell types during early neurogenesis of the mouse cerebellum. Elife. 2019 Feb 8;8:e42388. doi: 10.7554/eLife.42388. PMID: 30735127; PMCID: PMC6382353.

[62] Carter RA, Bihannic L, Rosencrance C, Hadley JL, Tong Y, Phoenix TN, Natarajan S, Easton J, Northcott PA, Gawad C. A Single-Cell Transcriptional Atlas of the Developing Murine Cerebellum. Curr Biol. 2018 Sep 24;28(18):2910-2920.e2. doi: 10.1016/j.cub.2018.07.062. Epub 2018 Sep 13. PMID: 30220501.

[63] Joyner AL. From Cloning Neural Development Genes to Functional Studies in Mice, 30 Years of Advancements. Curr Top Dev Biol. 2016;116:501-515. doi: 10.1016/bs.ctdb.2015.11.035. Epub 2016 Feb 17. PMID: 26970637.

[64] Rahimi-Balaei M, Bergen H, Kong J, Marzban H. Neuronal Migration During Development of the Cerebellum. Front Cell Neurosci. 2018a Dec 17;12:484. doi: 10.3389/fncel.2018.00484. PMID: 30618631; PMCID: PMC6304365.

[65] Sgaier SK, Millet S, Villanueva MP, Berenshteyn F, Song C, Joyner AL. Morphogenetic and cellular movements that shape the mouse cerebellum; insights from genetic fate mapping. Neuron. 2005 Jan 6;45(1):27-40. doi: 10.1016/j.neuron.2004.12.021. PMID: 15629700.

[66] Kratochwil CF, Maheshwari U, Rijli FM. The Long Journey of Pontine Nuclei Neurons: From Rhombic Lip to Cortico-Ponto-Cerebellar Circuitry. Front Neural Circuits. 2017 May 17;11:33. doi: 10.3389/fncir.2017.00033. PMID: 28567005; PMCID: PMC5434118.

[67] Florio M, Huttner WB. Neural progenitors, neurogenesis and the evolution of the neocortex. Development. 2014 Jun;141(11):2182-2194. doi: 10.1242/dev.090571. PMID: 24866113.

[68] Molnár Z, Pollen A. How unique is the human neocortex? Development. 2014 Jan;141(1):11-16. doi: 10.1242/dev.101279. PMID: 24346696.

[69] Nowakowski TJ, Bhaduri A, Pollen AA, Alvarado B, Mostajo-Radji MA, Di Lullo E, Haeussler M, Sandoval-Espinosa C, Liu SJ, Velmeshev D, Ounadjela JR, Shuga J, Wang X, Lim DA, West JA, Leyrat AA, Kent WJ, Kriegstein AR. Spatiotemporal gene expression trajectories reveal developmental hierarchies of the human cortex. Science. 2017 Dec 8;358(6368):1318-1323. doi: 10.1126/science.aap8809. PMID: 29217575; PMCID: PMC5991609.

[70] Eddison M, Toole L, Bell E, Wingate RJ. Segmental identity and

cerebellar granule cell induction in rhombomere 1. BMC Biol. 2004 Jun 15;2:14. doi: 10.1186/1741-7007-2-14. PMID: 15198802; PMCID: PMC446226.

[71] Garda AL, Echevarría D, Martínez S. Neuroepithelial co-expression of Gbx2 and Otx2 precedes Fgf8 expression in the isthmic organizer. Mech Dev. 2001 Mar;101(1-2):111-118. doi: 10.1016/s0925-4773(00)00567-0. PMID: 11231064.

[72] Hidalgo-Sánchez M, Millet S, Bloch-Gallego E, Alvarado-Mallart RM. Specification of the meso-isthmo-cerebellar region: the Otx2/Gbx2 boundary. Brain Res Brain Res Rev. 2005 Sep;49(2):134-149. doi: 10.1016/j.brainresrev.2005.01.010. Epub 2005 Mar 16. PMID: 16111544.

[73] McMahon AP, Bradley A. The Wnt-1 (int-1) proto-oncogene is required for development of a large region of the mouse brain. Cell. 1990a Sep 21;62(6):1073-1085. doi: 10.1016/0092-8674(90)90385-r. PMID: 2205396.

[74] Wurst W, Bally-Cuif L. Neural plate patterning: upstream and downstream of the isthmic organizer. Nat Rev Neurosci. 2001 Feb;2(2):99-108. doi: 10.1038/35053516. PMID: 11253000.

[75] Harada H, Sato T, Nakamura H. Fgf8 signaling for development of the midbrain and hindbrain. Dev Growth Differ. 2016 Jun;58(5):437-445. doi: 10.1111/dgd.12293. Epub 2016 Jun 7. PMID: 27273073.

[76] Mason I, Chambers D, Shamim H, Walshe J, Irving C. Regulation and function of FGF8 in patterning of midbrain and anterior hindbrain. Biochem Cell Biol. 2000;78(5):577-584. PMID: 11103948.

[77] Sato T, Joyner AL. The duration of Fgf8 isthmic organizer expression is key to patterning different tectal-isthmo-cerebellum structures. Development. 2009 Nov;136(21):3617-26. doi: 10.1242/dev.041210. Epub 2009 Sep 30. PMID: 19793884; PMCID: PMC2761110.

[78] Irving C, Mason I. Signalling by FGF8 from the isthmus patterns anterior hindbrain and establishes the anterior limit of Hox gene expression. Development. 2000 Jan;127(1):177-186. PMID: 10654611.

[79] Olander S, Nordström U, Patthey C, Edlund T. Convergent Wnt and FGF signaling at the gastrula stage induce the formation of the isthmic organizer. Mech Dev. 2006 Feb;123(2):166-176. doi: 10.1016/j.mod.2005.11.001. Epub 2006 Jan 18. PMID: 16413176.

[80] Chi CL, Martinez S, Wurst W, Martin GR. The isthmic organizer signal FGF8 is required for cell survival in the prospective midbrain and cerebellum. Development. 2003 Jun;130(12):2633-2644. doi: 10.1242/dev.00487. PMID: 12736208.

[81] Basson MA, Echevarria D, Ahn CP, Sudarov A, Joyner AL, Mason IJ, Martinez S, Martin GR. Specific regions within the embryonic midbrain and cerebellum require different levels of FGF signaling during development. Development. 2008 Mar;135(5):889-98. doi: 10.1242/dev.011569. Epub 2008 Jan 23. Erratum in: Development. 2009 Jun;136(11):1962. PMID: 18216176; PMCID: PMC2555978.

[82] Huang X, Liu J, Ketova T, Fleming JT, Grover VK, Cooper MK, Litingtung Y, Chiang C. Transventricular delivery of Sonic hedgehog is essential to cerebellar ventricular zone development. Proc Natl Acad Sci U S A. 2010 May 4;107(18):8422-7. doi: 10.1073/pnas.0911838107. Epub 2010 Apr 16. PMID: 20400693; PMCID: PMC2889567.

[83] Corrales JD, Rocco GL, Blaess S, Guo Q, Joyner AL. Spatial pattern of sonic hedgehog signaling through Gli genes during cerebellum development.

Development. 2004a Nov;131(22):5581-5590. doi: 10.1242/dev.01438. Epub 2004 Oct 20. PMID: 15496441.

[84] Millen KJ, Steshina EY, Iskusnykh IY, Chizhikov VV. Transformation of the cerebellum into more ventral brainstem fates causes cerebellar agenesis in the absence of Ptf1a function. Proc Natl Acad Sci U S A. 2014 Apr 29;111(17):E1777-86. doi: 10.1073/pnas.1315024111. Epub 2014 Apr 14. PMID: 24733890; PMCID: PMC4035921.

[85] Yamada M, Seto Y, Taya S, Owa T, Inoue YU, Inoue T, Kawaguchi Y, Nabeshima Y, Hoshino M. Specification of spatial identities of cerebellar neuron progenitors by ptf1a and atoh1 for proper production of GABAergic and glutamatergic neurons. J Neurosci. 2014 Apr 2;34(14):4786-800. doi: 10.1523/JNEUROSCI.2722-13.2014. PMID: 24695699; PMCID: PMC6802724.

[86] Seto Y, Nakatani T, Masuyama N, Taya S, Kumai M, Minaki Y, Hamaguchi A, Inoue YU, Inoue T, Miyashita S, Fujiyama T, Yamada M, Chapman H, Campbell K, Magnuson MA, Wright CV, Kawaguchi Y, Ikenaka K, Takebayashi H, Ishiwata S, Ono Y, Hoshino M. Temporal identity transition from Purkinje cell progenitors to GABAergic interneuron progenitors in the cerebellum. Nat Commun. 2014;5:3337. doi: 10.1038/ncomms4337. PMID: 24535035; PMCID: PMC5669625.

[87] Sudarov A, Turnbull RK, Kim EJ, Lebel-Potter M, Guillemot F, Joyner AL. Ascl1 genetics reveals insights into cerebellum local circuit assembly. J Neurosci. 2011 Jul 27;31(30):11055-69. doi: 10.1523/JNEUROSCI.0479-11.2011. PMID: 21795554; PMCID: PMC3153985.

[88] Hevner RF, Hodge RD, Daza RA, Englund C. Transcription factors in glutamatergic neurogenesis: conserved programs in neocortex, cerebellum, and adult hippocampus. Neurosci Res. 2006 Jul;55(3):223-233. doi: 10.1016/j.neures.2006.03.004. Epub 2006 Apr 18. PMID: 16621079.

[89] Haldipur P, Bharti U, Govindan S, Sarkar C, Iyengar S, Gressens P, Mani S. Expression of Sonic hedgehog during cell proliferation in the human cerebellum. Stem Cells Dev. 2012a May 1;21(7):1059-1068. doi: 10.1089/scd.2011.0206. Epub 2011 Aug 24. PMID: 21732818.

[90] Rakic P, Sidman RL. Histogenesis of cortical layers in human cerebellum, particularly the lamina dissecans. J Comp Neurol. 1970 Aug;139(4):473-500. doi: 10.1002/cne.901390407. PMID: 4195699.

[91] Zecevic N, Rakic P. Differentiation of Purkinje cells and their relationship to other components of developing cerebellar cortex in man. J Comp Neurol. 1976 May 1;167(1):27-47. doi: 10.1002/cne.901670103. PMID: 818132.

[92] Wefers AK, Haberlandt C, Surchev L, Steinhäuser C, Jabs R, Schilling K. Migration of Interneuron Precursors in the Nascent Cerebellar Cortex. Cerebellum. 2018 Feb;17(1):62-71. doi: 10.1007/s12311-017-0900-7. PMID: 29149443.

[93] Morales D, Hatten ME. Molecular markers of neuronal progenitors in the embryonic cerebellar anlage. J Neurosci. 2006 Nov 22;26(47):12226-36. doi: 10.1523/JNEUROSCI.3493-06.2006. PMID: 17122047; PMCID: PMC6675436.

[94] Dahmane N, Ruiz i Altaba A. Sonic hedgehog regulates the growth and patterning of the cerebellum. Development. 1999 Jun;126(14):3089-3100. PMID: 10375501.

[95] Solecki DJ, Liu XL, Tomoda T, Fang Y, Hatten ME. Activated Notch2 signaling inhibits differentiation of cerebellar granule neuron precursors by maintaining proliferation. Neuron. 2001 Aug 30;31(4):557-568.

doi: 10.1016/s0896-6273(01)00395-6. PMID: 11545715.

[96] Sudarov A, Joyner AL. Cerebellum morphogenesis: the foliation pattern is orchestrated by multi-cellular anchoring centers. Neural Dev. 2007 Dec 3;2:26. doi: 10.1186/1749-8104-2-26. PMID: 18053187; PMCID: PMC2246128.

[97] Cheng FY, Fleming JT, Chiang C. Bergmann glial Sonic hedgehog signaling activity is required for proper cerebellar cortical expansion and architecture. Dev Biol. 2018 Aug 15;440(2):152-166. doi: 10.1016/j.ydbio.2018.05.015. Epub 2018 May 21. PMID: 29792854; PMCID: PMC6014626.

[98] De Luca A, Parmigiani E, Tosatto G, Martire S, Hoshino M, Buffo A, Leto K, Rossi F. Exogenous Sonic hedgehog modulates the pool of GABAergic interneurons during cerebellar development. Cerebellum. 2015 Apr;14(2):72-85. doi: 10.1007/s12311-014-0596-x. PMID: 25245619.

[99] Hirai H, Launey T. The regulatory connection between the activity of granule cell NMDA receptors and dendritic differentiation of cerebellar Purkinje cells. J Neurosci. 2000 Jul 15;20(14):5217-24. doi: 10.1523/JNEUROSCI.20-14-05217.2000. PMID: 10884305; PMCID: PMC6772348.

[100] Ohashi R, Sakata S, Naito A, Hirashima N, Tanaka M. Dendritic differentiation of cerebellar Purkinje cells is promoted by ryanodine receptors expressed by Purkinje and granule cells. Dev Neurobiol. 2014 Apr;74(4):467-480. doi: 10.1002/dneu.22139. Epub 2013 Nov 4. PMID: 24123915.

[101] Xu X, Stoyanova EI, Lemiesz AE, Xing J, Mash DC, Heintz N. Species and cell-type properties of classically defined human and rodent neurons and glia. Elife. 2018 Oct 15;7:e37551. doi: 10.7554/eLife.37551. PMID: 30320555; PMCID: PMC6188473.

[102] Peng J, Sheng AL, Xiao Q, Shen L, Ju XC, Zhang M, He ST, Wu C, Luo ZG. Single-cell transcriptomes reveal molecular specializations of neuronal cell types in the developing cerebellum. J Mol Cell Biol. 2019 Aug 19;11(8):636-648. doi: 10.1093/jmcb/mjy089. PMID: 30690467; PMCID: PMC6788728.

[103] Watanabe K, Kamiya D, Nishiyama A, Katayama T, Nozaki S, Kawasaki H, Watanabe Y, Mizuseki K, Sasai Y. Directed differentiation of telencephalic precursors from embryonic stem cells. Nat Neurosci. 2005 Mar;8(3):288-296. doi: 10.1038/nn1402. Epub 2005 Feb 6. PMID: 15696161.

[104] Elkabetz Y, Panagiotakos G, Al Shamy G, Socci ND, Tabar V, Studer L. Human ES cell-derived neural rosettes reveal a functionally distinct early neural stem cell stage. Genes Dev. 2008 Jan 15;22(2):152-65. doi: 10.1101/gad.1616208. Erratum in: Genes Dev. 2008 May 1;22(9):1257. PMID: 18198334; PMCID: PMC2192751.

[105] Koch P, Opitz T, Steinbeck JA, Ladewig J, Brüstle O. A rosette-type, self-renewing human ES cell-derived neural stem cell with potential for in vitro instruction and synaptic integration. Proc Natl Acad Sci U S A. 2009 Mar 3;106(9):3225-30. doi: 10.1073/pnas.0808387106. Epub 2009 Feb 13. PMID: 19218428; PMCID: PMC2651316.

[106] Eiraku M, Watanabe K, Matsuo-Takasaki M, Kawada M, Yonemura S, Matsumura M, Wataya T, Nishiyama A, Muguruma K, Sasai Y. Self-organized formation of polarized cortical tissues from ESCs and its active manipulation by extrinsic signals. Cell Stem Cell. 2008 Nov 6;3(5):519-532. doi: 10.1016/j.stem.2008.09.002. PMID: 18983967.

[107] Bavassano C, Eigentler A, Stanika R, Obermair GJ, Boesch S,

Dechant G, Nat R. Bicistronic CACNA1A Gene Expression in Neurons Derived from Spinocerebellar Ataxia Type 6 Patient-Induced Pluripotent Stem Cells. Stem Cells Dev. 2017 Nov 15;26(22):1612-1625. doi: 10.1089/scd.2017.0085. Epub 2017 Oct 30. PMID: 28946818; PMCID: PMC5684673.

[108] Zhou S, Ochalek A, Szczesna K, Avci HX, Kobolák J, Varga E, Rasmussen M, Holst B, Cirera S, Hyttel P, Freude KK, Dinnyés A. The positional identity of iPSC-derived neural progenitor cells along the anterior-posterior axis is controlled in a dosage-dependent manner by bFGF and EGF. Differentiation. 2016 Oct-Nov;92(4):183-194. doi: 10.1016/j.diff.2016.06.002. Epub 2016 Jun 16. PMID: 27321088.

[109] Rifes P, Isaksson M, Rathore GS, Aldrin-Kirk P, Møller OK, Barzaghi G, Lee J, Egerod KL, Rausch DM, Parmar M, Pers TH, Laurell T, Kirkeby A. Modeling neural tube development by differentiation of human embryonic stem cells in a microfluidic WNT gradient. Nat Biotechnol. 2020 Nov;38(11):1265-1273. doi: 10.1038/s41587-020-0525-0. Epub 2020 May 25. Erratum in: Nat Biotechnol. 2020 Jun 11;: PMID: 32451506.

[110] Kirkeby A, Nelander J, Parmar M. Generating regionalized neuronal cells from pluripotency, a step-by-step protocol. Front Cell Neurosci. 2013 Jan 3;6:64. doi: 10.3389/fncel.2012.00064. PMID: 23316134; PMCID: PMC3539732.

[111] Tailor J, Kittappa R, Leto K, Gates M, Borel M, Paulsen O, Spitzer S, Karadottir RT, Rossi F, Falk A, Smith A. Stem cells expanded from the human embryonic hindbrain stably retain regional specification and high neurogenic potency. J Neurosci. 2013 Jul 24;33(30):12407-22. doi: 10.1523/JNEUROSCI.0130-13.2013. PMID: 23884946; PMCID: PMC3721847.

[112] Johnson MA, Weick JP, Pearce RA, Zhang SC. Functional neural development from human embryonic stem cells: accelerated synaptic activity via astrocyte coculture. J Neurosci. 2007 Mar 21;27(12):3069-77. doi: 10.1523/JNEUROSCI.4562-06.2007. PMID: 17376968; PMCID: PMC2735200.

[113] Murrow LM, Weber RJ, Gartner ZJ. Dissecting the stem cell niche with organoid models: an engineering-based approach. Development. 2017 Mar 15;144(6):998-1007. doi: 10.1242/dev.140905. PMID: 28292846; PMCID: PMC5358107.

[114] He L, Zhao H, Li S, Han X, Chen Z, Wang C, Tian C, Tang F, Huang R, Lin Z, Li Z, Tang B, Jiang H. Generation of induced pluripotent stem cell line (CSUXHi002-A) from a patient with spinocerebellar ataxia type 1. Stem Cell Res. 2020 May;45:101816. doi: 10.1016/j.scr.2020.101816. Epub 2020 Apr 21. PMID: 32335388.

[115] Buijsen RAM, Gardiner SL, Bouma MJ, van der Graaf LM, Boogaard MW, Pepers BA, Eussen B, de Klein A, Freund C, van Roon-Mom WMC. Generation of 3 spinocerebellar ataxia type 1 (SCA1) patient-derived induced pluripotent stem cell lines LUMCi002-A, B, and C and 2 unaffected sibling control induced pluripotent stem cell lines LUMCi003-A and B. Stem Cell Res. 2018 May;29:125-128. doi: 10.1016/j.scr.2018.03.018. Epub 2018 Apr 5. PMID: 29656178.

[116] Xia G, Santostefano K, Hamazaki T, Liu J, Subramony SH, Terada N, Ashizawa T. Generation of human-induced pluripotent stem cells to model spinocerebellar ataxia type 2 in vitro. J Mol Neurosci. 2013 Oct;51(2):237-48. doi: 10.1007/s12031-012-9930-2. Epub 2012 Dec 9. PMID: 23224816; PMCID: PMC3608734.

[117] Chuang CY, Yang CC, Soong BW, Yu CY, Chen SH, Huang HP, Kuo HC.

Modeling spinocerebellar ataxias 2 and 3 with iPSCs reveals a role for glutamate in disease pathology. Sci Rep. 2019 Feb 4;9(1):1166. doi: 10.1038/s41598-018-37774-2. PMID: 30718627; PMCID: PMC6361947.

[118] Koch P, Breuer P, Peitz M, Jungverdorben J, Kesavan J, Poppe D, Doerr J, Ladewig J, Mertens J, Tüting T, Hoffmann P, Klockgether T, Evert BO, Wüllner U, Brüstle O. Excitation-induced ataxin-3 aggregation in neurons from patients with Machado-Joseph disease. Nature. 2011 Nov 23;480(7378):543-6. doi: 10.1038/nature10671. PMID: 22113611.

[119] Moore LR, Keller L, Bushart DD, Delatorre RG, Li D, McLoughlin HS, do Carmo Costa M, Shakkottai VG, Smith GD, Paulson HL. Antisense oligonucleotide therapy rescues aggresome formation in a novel spinocerebellar ataxia type 3 human embryonic stem cell line. Stem Cell Res. 2019 Aug;39:101504. doi: 10.1016/j.scr.2019.101504. Epub 2019 Jul 16. PMID: 31374463; PMCID: PMC6736695.

[120] Hansen SK, Stummann TC, Borland H, Hasholt LF, Tümer Z, Nielsen JE, Rasmussen MA, Nielsen TT, Daechsel JC, Fog K, Hyttel P. Induced pluripotent stem cell - derived neurons for the study of spinocerebellar ataxia type 3. Stem Cell Res. 2016 Sep;17(2):306-317. doi: 10.1016/j.scr.2016.07.004. Epub 2016 Aug 16. PMID: 27596958.

[121] Ou Z, Luo M, Niu X, Chen Y, Xie Y, He W, Song B, Xian Y, Fan D, OuYang S, Sun X. Autophagy Promoted the Degradation of Mutant ATXN3 in Neurally Differentiated Spinocerebellar Ataxia-3 Human Induced Pluripotent Stem Cells. Biomed Res Int. 2016;2016:6701793. doi: 10.1155/2016/6701793. Epub 2016 Oct 25. PMID: 27847820; PMCID: PMC5099487.

[122] Ouyang S, Xie Y, Xiong Z, Yang Y, Xian Y, Ou Z, Song B, Chen Y, Xie Y, Li H, Sun X. CRISPR/Cas9-Targeted Deletion of Polyglutamine in Spinocerebellar Ataxia Type 3-Derived Induced Pluripotent Stem Cells. Stem Cells Dev. 2018 Jun 1;27(11):756-770. doi: 10.1089/scd.2017.0209. Epub 2018 May 18. PMID: 29661116.

[123] Luo Y, Fan Y, Zhou B, Xu Z, Chen Y, Sun X. Generation of induced pluripotent stem cells from skin fibroblasts of a patient with olivopontocerebellar atrophy. Tohoku J Exp Med. 2012 Feb;226(2):151-9. doi: 10.1620/tjem.226.151. PMID: 22301348.

[124] Ward JM, Stoyas CA, Switonski PM, Ichou F, Fan W, Collins B, Wall CE, Adanyeguh I, Niu C, Sopher BL, Kinoshita C, Morrison RS, Durr A, Muotri AR, Evans RM, Mochel F, La Spada AR. Metabolic and Organelle Morphology Defects in Mice and Human Patients Define Spinocerebellar Ataxia Type 7 as a Mitochondrial Disease. Cell Rep. 2019 Jan 29;26(5):1189-1202.e6. doi: 10.1016/j.celrep.2019.01.028. PMID: 30699348; PMCID: PMC6420346.

[125] Kumar D, Hussain A, Srivastava AK, Mukerji M, Mukherjee O, Faruq M. Generation of three spinocerebellar ataxia type-12 patients derived induced pluripotent stem cell lines (IGIBi002-A, IGIBi003-A and IGIBi004-A). Stem Cell Res. 2018 Aug;31:216-221. doi: 10.1016/j.scr.2018.08.008.

[126] Matsuzono K, Imamura K, Murakami N, Tsukita K, Yamamoto T, Izumi Y, Kaji R, Ohta Y, Yamashita T, Abe K, Inoue H. Antisense Oligonucleotides Reduce RNA Foci in Spinocerebellar Ataxia 36 Patient iPSCs. Mol Ther Nucleic Acids. 2017 Sep 15;8:211-219. doi: 10.1016/j.omtn.2017.06.017. Epub 2017 Jun 23. PMID: 28918022; PMCID: PMC5504081.

[127] Morino H, Matsuda Y, Muguruma K, Miyamoto R, Ohsawa R, Ohtake T,

Otobe R, Watanabe M, Maruyama H, Hashimoto K, Kawakami H. A mutation in the low voltage-gated calcium channel CACNA1G alters the physiological properties of the channel, causing spinocerebellar ataxia. Mol Brain. 2015 Dec 29;8:89. doi: 10.1186/s13041-015-0180-4. PMID: 26715324; PMCID: PMC4693440.

[128] Eigentler A, Boesch S, Schneider R, Dechant G, Nat R. Induced pluripotent stem cells from friedreich ataxia patients fail to upregulate frataxin during in vitro differentiation to peripheral sensory neurons. Stem Cells Dev. 2013 Dec 15;22(24):3271-3282. doi: 10.1089/scd.2013.0126. Epub 2013 Aug 24. PMID: 23879205.

[129] Lai JI, Nachun D, Petrosyan L, Throesch B, Campau E, Gao F, Baldwin KK, Coppola G, Gottesfeld JM, Soragni E. Transcriptional profiling of isogenic Friedreich ataxia neurons and effect of an HDAC inhibitor on disease signatures. J Biol Chem. 2019 Feb 8;294(6):1846-1859. doi: 10.1074/jbc.RA118.006515

[130] Ku S, Soragni E, Campau E, Thomas EA, Altun G, Laurent LC, Loring JF, Napierala M, Gottesfeld JM. Friedreich's ataxia induced pluripotent stem cells model intergenerational GAA·TTC triplet repeat instability. Cell Stem Cell. 2010 Nov 5;7(5):631-7. doi: 10.1016/j.stem.2010.09.014. PMID: 21040903; PMCID: PMC2987635.

[131] Polak U, Li Y, Butler JS, Napierala M. Alleviating GAA Repeat Induced Transcriptional Silencing of the Friedreich's Ataxia Gene During Somatic Cell Reprogramming. Stem Cells Dev. 2016 Dec 1;25(23):1788-1800. doi: 10.1089/scd.2016.0147. Epub 2016 Oct 17. PMID: 27615158; PMCID: PMC5155629.

[132] Bird MJ, Needham K, Frazier AE, van Rooijen J, Leung J, Hough S, Denham M, Thornton ME, Parish CL, Nayagam BA, Pera M, Thorburn DR, Thompson LH, Dottori M. Functional characterization of Friedreich ataxia iPS-derived neuronal progenitors and their integration in the adult brain. PLoS One. 2014 Jul 7;9(7):e101718. doi: 10.1371/journal.pone.0101718. PMID: 25000412; PMCID: PMC4084949.

[133] Hick A, Wattenhofer-Donzé M, Chintawar S, Tropel P, Simard JP, Vaucamps N, Gall D, Lambot L, André C, Reutenauer L, Rai M, Teletin M, Messaddeq N, Schiffmann SN, Viville S, Pearson CE, Pandolfo M, Puccio H. Neurons and cardiomyocytes derived from induced pluripotent stem cells as a model for mitochondrial defects in Friedreich's ataxia. Dis Model Mech. 2013 May;6(3):608-21. doi: 10.1242/dmm.010900. Epub 2012 Nov 7. PMID: 23136396; PMCID: PMC3634645.

[134] Mazzara PG, Muggeo S, Luoni M, Massimino L, Zaghi M, Valverde PT, Brusco S, Marzi MJ, Palma C, Colasante G, Iannielli A, Paulis M, Cordiglieri C, Giannelli SG, Podini P, Gellera C, Taroni F, Nicassio F, Rasponi M, Broccoli V. Frataxin gene editing rescues Friedreich's ataxia pathology in dorsal root ganglia organoid-derived sensory neurons. Nat Commun. 2020 Aug 21;11(1):4178. doi: 10.1038/s41467-020-17954-3. PMID: 32826895; PMCID: PMC7442818.

[135] Nayler SP, Powell JE, Vanichkina DP, Korn O, Wells CA, Kanjhan R, Sun J, Taft RJ, Lavin MF, Wolvetang EJ. Human iPSC-Derived Cerebellar Neurons from a Patient with Ataxia-Telangiectasia Reveal Disrupted Gene Regulatory Networks. Front Cell Neurosci. 2017 Oct 13;11:321. doi: 10.3389/fncel.2017.00321. PMID: 29081736; PMCID: PMC5645492.

[136] Rüb U, Schöls L, Paulson H, Auburger G, Kermer P, Jen JC, Seidel K, Korf HW, Deller T. Clinical features, neurogenetics and neuropathology

of the polyglutamine spinocerebellar ataxias type 1, 2, 3, 6 and 7. Prog Neurobiol. 2013 May;104:38-66. doi: 10.1016/j.pneurobio.2013.01.001. Epub 2013 Feb 21. PMID: 23438480.

[137] Seidel K, Siswanto S, Brunt ER, den Dunnen W, Korf HW, Rüb U. Brain pathology of spinocerebellar ataxias. Acta Neuropathol. 2012 Jul;124(1):1-21. doi: 10.1007/s00401-012-1000-x. Epub 2012 Jun 9. PMID: 22684686.

[138] Sullivan R, Yau WY, O'Connor E, Houlden H. Spinocerebellar ataxia: an update. J Neurol. 2019 Feb;266(2):533-544. doi: 10.1007/s00415-018-9076-4. Epub 2018 Oct 3. PMID: 30284037; PMCID: PMC6373366.

[139] Choy KR, Watters DJ. Neurodegeneration in ataxia-telangiectasia: Multiple roles of ATM kinase in cellular homeostasis. Dev Dyn. 2018 Jan;247(1):33-46. doi: 10.1002/dvdy.24522. Epub 2017 Jun 5. PMID: 28543935.

[140] Robinson KJ, Watchon M, Laird AS. Aberrant Cerebellar Circuitry in the Spinocerebellar Ataxias. Front Neurosci. 2020 Jul 16;14:707. doi: 10.3389/fnins.2020.00707. PMID: 32765211; PMCID: PMC7378801.

[141] Solodkin, A. and Gomez, C.M., (2012). Spinocerebellar ataxia type 6. Handb. Clin. Neurol. *103*, 461-473.

[142] Tada M, Nishizawa M, Onodera O. Redefining cerebellar ataxia in degenerative ataxias: lessons from recent research on cerebellar systems. J Neurol Neurosurg Psychiatry. 2015 Aug;86(8):922-928. doi: 10.1136/jnnp-2013-307225. Epub 2015 Jan 30. PMID: 25637456.

[143] Fan HC, Ho LI, Chi CS, Chen SJ, Peng GS, Chan TM, Lin SZ, Harn HJ. Polyglutamine (PolyQ) diseases: genetics to treatments. Cell Transplant. 2014;23(4-5):441-458. doi: 10.3727/096368914X678454. PMID: 24816443.

[144] La Spada AR, Taylor JP. Repeat expansion disease: progress and puzzles in disease pathogenesis. Nat Rev Genet. 2010 Apr;11(4):247-58. doi: 10.1038/nrg2748. PMID: 20177426; PMCID: PMC4704680.

[145] Orr HT, Zoghbi HY. Trinucleotide repeat disorders. Annu Rev Neurosci. 2007;30:575-621. doi: 10.1146/annurev.neuro.29.051605.113042. PMID: 17417937.

[146] Cohen-Carmon D, Meshorer E. Polyglutamine (polyQ) disorders: the chromatin connection. Nucleus. 2012 Sep-Oct;3(5):433-41. doi: 10.4161/nucl.21481. Epub 2012 Aug 15. PMID: 22892726; PMCID: PMC3474664.

[147] Tezenas du Montcel S, Durr A, Bauer P, Figueroa KP, Ichikawa Y, Brussino A, Forlani S, Rakowicz M, Schöls L, Mariotti C, van de Warrenburg BP, Orsi L, Giunti P, Filla A, Szymanski S, Klockgether T, Berciano J, Pandolfo M, Boesch S, Melegh B, Timmann D, Mandich P, Camuzat A; Clinical Research Consortium for Spinocerebellar Ataxia (CRC-SCA); EUROSCA network, Goto J, Ashizawa T, Cazeneuve C, Tsuji S, Pulst SM, Brusco A, Riess O, Brice A, Stevanin G. Modulation of the age at onset in spinocerebellar ataxia by CAG tracts in various genes. Brain. 2014 Sep;137(Pt 9):2444-55. doi: 10.1093/brain/awu174. Epub 2014 Jun 26. PMID: 24972706; PMCID: PMC4132646.

[148] Ashizawa T, Öz G, Paulson HL. Spinocerebellar ataxias: prospects and challenges for therapy development. Nat Rev Neurol. 2018 Oct;14(10):590-605. doi: 10.1038/s41582-018-0051-6. Erratum in: Nat Rev Neurol. 2018 Dec;14(12):749. PMID: 30131520; PMCID: PMC6469934.

[149] Shum, C. and Nishimura, A.L., (2015). iPS Cells and Spinocerebellar Ataxia. In *Stem Cells in Modeling Human Genetic Diseases*, M. Zatz, and O. Keith Okamoto, eds. Springer International Publishing, pp. 45-61.

[150] Du X, Wang J, Zhu H, Rinaldo L, Lamar KM, Palmenberg AC, Hansel C, Gomez CM. Second cistron in CACNA1A gene encodes a transcription factor mediating cerebellar development and SCA6. Cell. 2013 Jul 3;154(1):118-33. doi: 10.1016/j.cell.2013.05.059. PMID: 23827678; PMCID: PMC3939801.

[151] Garden GA, La Spada AR. Molecular pathogenesis and cellular pathology of spinocerebellar ataxia type 7 neurodegeneration. Cerebellum. 2008;7(2):138-49. doi: 10.1007/s12311-008-0027-y. PMID: 18418675; PMCID: PMC4195584.

[152] Fogel BL, Perlman S. Clinical features and molecular genetics of autosomal recessive cerebellar ataxias. Lancet Neurol. 2007 Mar;6(3):245-257. doi: 10.1016/S1474-4422(07)70054-6. PMID: 17303531.

[153] Synofzik M, Puccio H, Mochel F, Schöls L. Autosomal Recessive Cerebellar Ataxias: Paving the Way toward Targeted Molecular Therapies. Neuron. 2019 Feb 20;101(4):560-583. doi: 10.1016/j.neuron.2019.01.049. PMID: 30790538.

[154] Lim J, Hao T, Shaw C, Patel AJ, Szabó G, Rual JF, Fisk CJ, Li N, Smolyar A, Hill DE, Barabási AL, Vidal M, Zoghbi HY. A protein-protein interaction network for human inherited ataxias and disorders of Purkinje cell degeneration. Cell. 2006 May 19;125(4):801-814. doi: 10.1016/j.cell.2006.03.032. PMID: 16713569.

[155] Cohen-Carmon D, Sorek M, Lerner V, Divya MS, Nissim-Rafinia M, Yarom Y, Meshorer E. Progerin-Induced Transcriptional Changes in Huntington's Disease Human Pluripotent Stem Cell-Derived Neurons. Mol Neurobiol. 2020 Mar;57(3):1768-1777. PMID: 31939145.

[156] Miller JD, Ganat YM, Kishinevsky S, Bowman RL, Liu B, Tu EY, Mandal PK, Vera E, Shim JW, Kriks S, Taldone T, Fusaki N, Tomishima MJ, Krainc D, Milner TA, Rossi DJ, Studer L. Human iPSC-based modeling of late-onset disease via progerin-induced aging. Cell Stem Cell. 2013 Dec 5;13(6):691-705. doi: 10.1016/j.stem.2013.11.006. PMID: 24315443; PMCID: PMC4153390.

[157] Tamada A, Watanabe S, Muguruma K. Investigating developmental and disease mechanisms of the cerebellum with pluripotent stem cells. Mol Cell Neurosci. 2020 Sep;107:103530. doi: 10.1016/j.mcn.2020.103530. Epub 2020 Jul 18. PMID: 32693017.

[158] Cornacchia D, Studer L. Back and forth in time: Directing age in iPSC-derived lineages. Brain Res. 2017a Feb 1;1656:14-26. doi: 10.1016/j.brainres.2015.11.013. Epub 2015 Nov 17. PMID: 26592774; PMCID: PMC4870156.

[159] Bettencourt C, Ryten M, Forabosco P, Schorge S, Hersheson J, Hardy J, Houlden H; United Kingdom Brain Expression Consortium. Insights from cerebellar transcriptomic analysis into the pathogenesis of ataxia. JAMA Neurol. 2014 Jul 1;71(7):831-9. doi: 10.1001/jamaneurol.2014.756. PMID: 24862029; PMCID: PMC4469030.

[160] Adli M. The CRISPR tool kit for genome editing and beyond. Nat Commun. 2018 May 15;9(1):1911. doi: 10.1038/s41467-018-04252-2. PMID: 29765029; PMCID: PMC5953931.

Chapter 5

Rehabilitation for Spinocerebellar Ataxia

Akiyoshi Matsugi, Kyota Bando, Yutaka Kikuchi, Yuki Kondo and Hideki Nakano

Abstract

Rehabilitation is an important treatment for spinocerebellar ataxia (SCA). The lack of improvement in ataxia, deficit of motor learning, and unstable balance causes disability for activities of daily living and restricts participation in social activities, further resulting in a disturbance of the restoration of quality of life. This narrative review describes physical rehabilitation, including measurement of movement disorder, associated with ataxia and possible interventions. Several lines of evidence suggest that high-intensity individualized physical rehabilitation programs, especially for gait and balance training, improve motor function. Continuous exercise at home contributes to the maintenance of the gait and balance function. Moreover, videography and mechanical technology contribute to the evaluation of ataxia and motor learning ability, and assistive robotic systems may improve gait stability. Neuromodulation montages, such as repetitive transcranial magnetic stimulation and transcranial electrical stimulation, can enhance the effect of physical rehabilitation. Further research aimed at developing a more-effective physical rehabilitation for these patients is expected.

Keywords: spinocerebellar ataxia, rehabilitation, physical therapy, ataxia, assessment, gait training, balance training, motor learning, assistive technology, neuromodulation, noninvasive brain stimulation

1. Introduction

Spinocerebellar ataxia (SCA), which is included in spinocerebellar degeneration (SCD), is a genetically heterogeneous group of autosomal dominantly inherited progressive disorders [1]. Cerebellar atrophy is the most prominent clinical feature of this condition and is accompanied by spinal cord and sequential brain stem and basal ganglion damage. Therefore, coordinated movement of the eyes, head, trunk, and extremities is impaired. Therefore, the activities of daily living (ADL) and participation in social activities are limited, and the quality of life (QOL) is undisputedly impaired in these patients [2].

The effects of medication and surgery in this clinical setting depend on the cause of ataxia and the extent of neuronal damage [3, 4]; however, there is no rational effective treatment for SCA and it is difficult to slow the progression of the disease. Rehabilitation [5, 6], including physical therapy [7, 8], aimed at improving/maintaining motor function, ADL, and QOL [5] is an important intervention for patients with SCA. Here we provide a narrative review of physical rehabilitation for SCA.

2. General features

For the clinical diagnosis of cerebellar ataxia, specific blood studies and magnetic resonance imaging (MRI) have been performed [9]. Furthermore, genetic techniques improve the diagnosis of degenerative cerebellar ataxia [10]. Although the details of the findings of these genetic and blood studies are beyond the scope of this review of rehabilitation, cerebellar atrophy and cerebellar motor deficits are traditionally common observations in patients with degenerative cerebellar ataxia [9]. Furthermore, recently, the absence of motor cerebellar symptoms has also been recognized as being important for rehabilitation [11].

The cerebellum is the motor-control system in humans [12]. Clinically, the oculomotor deficit, speech deficits, ataxia in the trunk and extremities, balance disorder, and gait disturbance are the targets of rehabilitation in SCA [9, 13]. The possible underlying pathogenetic mechanisms include distorted timing, abnormal sensory acquisition, impaired sensory motor synchronization, impaired triggering of corticomotor excitability, and abnormal visuokinesthetic cerebro-cerebellar interactions [13].

Oculomotor deficits cause deoptimized vision. The vestibulo-ocular reflex and smooth pursuit [14] partially depend on motor prediction in static and dynamic movement and contribute to dynamic gazing [15]; moreover, the cerebellum contributes to the trainability of eye-head coordinated movements [16].

Abnormal excitability and modulation in the motor cortex and corticospinal tract causes a voluntary contraction deficit in [17, 18]. Cerebellar stimulation modulates the motor-evoked potential induced by transcranial magnetic stimulation (TMS) of the primary motor cortex [19–21]; however, this modulation is absent in patients with SCA [22, 23]. Furthermore, the cortical silent period, which reflects the excitability of the inhibitory GABAergic neural circuit in the primary motor cortex, is abnormal in these patients [24–29], and this cerebellar effect on the cortical silent period is characteristic of the healthy population [30]. Before muscle contraction for movement, the corticospinal excitability increases in healthy individuals; in contrast, this facilitation is insufficient in SCA [31]. In addition, in patients with SCA, muscle tones are decreased [11] and the spinal reflex excitability is facilitated by cerebellar stimulation [32–34]. The long latency spinal reflex, which is correlated with the cortical circuit, is disturbed in SCA [35]. Although this functional cerebellum-spine connection may contribute to the preparation for muscle contraction, there is insufficient evidence that these connections contribute to motor control in healthy and cerebellar ataxia populations.

In simple movements, such as extension of the elbow, coordinated activity of the biceps and triceps is needed. For ballistic elbow-extension movement practice, the triphasic muscle agonist and antagonist contraction patterns contribute to the smooth movement, but under/overshooting appears during the uncoordinated contraction pattern of patients with SCA [36, 37]. Furthermore, this contraction pattern may be obtained by temporal electrical stimulation in these individuals [37].

The cerebellar internal model contributes to predictable/online/offline motor control and motor learning/adaptation [38]. The symptoms associated with motor learning do not appear at the onset of the cerebral atrophy [39], because several brain areas, i.e., the prefrontal cortex, primary motor cortex, and basal ganglia, compensate for cerebellar function in early-stage SCA [5, 6, 39]. Recently, the motor learning deficit at the early stage of the disorder was reportedly detected using an adaptation task [40]. Therefore, the assessment of the capacity for motor learning may be important to strategize the interventions that are concretely described in the following sections.

Representative nonataxia symptoms include hyperreflexia, areflexia, extensor plantar, spasticity, paresis, muscle atrophy, fasciculations, myoclonus, rigidity, chorea/dyskinesia, dystonia, resting tremor, sensory symptoms, urinary dysfunction, cognitive impairment, and brain stem oculomotor signs [41]. The Inventory of NonAtaxia Symptoms (INAS) [41] is used to estimate these nonataxia symptoms. The appearance of these symptoms depends on the type of SCA [41].

3. Assessment format

We should conduct assessment to detect the degree of motor dysfunction and consider more effective intervention of physical rehabilitation. The first, the imaging technology such as MRI provides us with structural information about the atrophic areas of the brain associated with the disease. We described about neuroimaging technique in Section 3.1. The next, we can use some outcome measurement to estimate the motor dysfunction and verification in the physical rehabilitation. Then, we introduce the representable outcome measures for physical rehabilitation in SCA in Section 3.2. However, we had not established method to estimate the remaining of motor learning ability, which is one of the most important factors to predict the effect of physical rehabilitation. Therefore, we propose the possible assessment of motor learning ability in Section 3.3.

3.1 Neuroimaging

Neuroimaging is a technique that is used to visualize the structural and functional activities of the brain. MRI measurements, such as diffusion tensor imaging and surface-based morphometry, visualize the brain structures. Functional activity imaging is achieved using fMRI and NIRS, which are indicators of cerebral blood flow, and electroencephalogram (EEG) and magnetoencephalography, which are indicators of electrical activity. Positron emission tomography and single-photon emission computed tomography with nuclear tracers are also used in this setting. The application of neuroimaging in the rehabilitation of cerebellar disorders includes voxel-based lesion symptom mapping in patients with stroke, to investigate the recovery of upper arm reach [42] and walking ability [43] depending on the lesion site.

Although conventional MRI [44] is widely used for the neuroimaging of spinocerebellar degeneration, to obtain diagnostic findings, few studies have used neuroimaging as a guideline or outcome of rehabilitation. The lack of reports in this context hampers the quantification of cerebellar degeneration in SCA and its correlation with motor dysfunctions. In terms of measurement techniques, the cerebellum exhibits a much tighter folding compared with the cerebral cortex, with individual cortical sheets with a thickness of 1–2 mm and a sheet area of 1500–2000 cm^2, compared with a sheet area of 2200 cm^2 with a thickness of 1.5–4 mm in the cerebral cortex. Therefore, the typical 2–4 mm^3 spatial resolution of neuroimaging techniques is insufficient to capture local cerebellar changes. Patient factors include the difficulty in limiting the brain regions involved in movement disorders to the cerebellum, because the degenerative regions in SCD extend beyond this structure to multiple brain regions [45].

Among the neuroimaging modalities, the role of voxel-based morphometry (VBM) is notable in SCA rehabilitation. VBM is a statistical analysis of the entire brain in voxel units (1 mm^3) that is used to identify the behavioral patterns and related brain morphological characteristics of patients [46]. Burciu et al. assessed the degree of cerebellar atrophy concerning motor and learning functions using VBM to evaluate brain structure changes after 2 weeks of balance training in patients with SCD; these authors reported the association between an increased volume of the dorsal premotor cortex and increased balance ability [47]. Matsgi et al. reported an association between VBM and neurophysiological markers in cerebellar brain inhibition (CBI), with atrophy of the dentate nucleus at VBM observed in cases of pure cerebellar ataxia that did not show CBI [48]. Bando et al. reported a correlation between adaptive learning ability and gray matter volume of the cerebellar IV-VII lobules and the supramarginal gyrus in a prismatic adaptation task in SCA [49]. Thus, VBM may be a biomarker to explain motor dysfunction in patients with SCA.

Conversely, VBM is not an ideal tool to show a causal relationship between brain structural changes and behavioral differences. As a solution to this problem, we can propose a combination of VBM and neurostimulation [50], as neurostimulation of the brain regions associated with the behavioral patterns obtained by VBM and the observation of behavioral changes before and after stimulation allow us to examine brain degeneration sites and behavior.

3.2 Outcome measurement

Gait disturbance is a major symptom of the cerebellar pathology in SCA [51]. The functional ambulation categories (FAC) is useful for the comprehensive assessment of walking ability; the FAC assesses gait for about 15 m and climbing stairs and classifies gait levels into 6 levels [52]. The FAC is also used in the exercise program created by Research Committee for Ataxia Disease (Research team under the jurisdiction of the Ministry of Health, Labour and Welfare in Japan, http://ataxia.umin.ne.jp/rehabilitation/).

The quantitative assessment of cerebellar ataxia is very important in clinical practice. The International Cooperative Ataxia Rating Scale (ICARS) has been used as a quantitative assessment of ataxia symptoms. However, it has been noted that the test reliability of the eye movement items is low [53]. The Scale for Assessment and Rating of Ataxia (SARA) is an 8-item performance-based scale that yields a total score of 0–40 (most severe ataxia). The minimal detectable change (MDC) for individual score difference from the baseline to the 1-year follow-up in SARA was <3.5 (n = 171; SCA1, n = 43; SCA2, n = 61; SCA3, n = 37; and SCA6, n = 30; mean age, 50.9 ± 13.5 years; mean disease duration, 11.8 ± 5.6 years) [54]. SARA does not include an eye movement section. Schmahmann et al. noted the importance of assessing oculomotor abnormalities and developed the Brief Ataxia Rating Scale, a modification of ICARS [55]. Each SCA genotype exhibits specific symptoms [56]. Therefore, these assessments should be used differently for different symptoms. However, one feature that is consistent among these assessments is that the scoring range is large and does not allow the assessment of minute symptom changes. Honda et al. developed a system to measure the evaluation of SARA using a depth sensor [57]. Using this system, the degree of ataxia can be measured numerically. In addition, because the system is inexpensive, it can be installed at the patient's home, making it a useful tool for telemedicine.

The balance dysfunction in SCA has a significant impact on QOL [58]. The Berg Balance Scale and the Timed Up and Go test are widely used to assess balance dysfunction in SCA [59]. However, despite their widespread use, these assessments have not been examined for reliability and validity in SCA. Kondo et al. examined the test reliability of the Balance Evaluation Systems Test (BESTest) [60]. The BESTest is a multitask balance assessment tool that was developed to identify specific postural control problems (i.e., biomechanical constraints, stability limits, anticipatory postural adjustments, postural responses, sensory orientation, dynamic balance during gait, and cognitive effects) [61]. The MDC for an individual score difference from the baseline to the 4-week follow-up in

BESTest was <8.7 (n = 20; SCA3, n = 4; SCA6, n = 9; SCA31, n = 7; mean age, 63.7 ± 10.1 years; age at onset, 53.9 ± 10.5 years; baseline SARA, 9.9 ± 3.5) [61]. Many types of balance function measures have been reported. However, BESTest is the only scale that is considered to have absolute reliability in SCA.

Gait speed is often used as an outcome of intervention studies in SCA [62, 63]. However, some changes in the gait pattern (e.g., base of support and gait speed) most likely reflect cerebellar-unspecific, compensatory strategies, and a high spatiotemporal gait variability appears to be a distinctive feature of ataxic gait [58, 64]. The Gait Variability Index (GVI) is a measure of gait variability that has been examined regarding reliability and validity [65]. The MDC for an individual score difference from day 1 to day 2 in GVI was <8.6 (Friedreich's ataxia, n = 81; baseline ICARS, 70.4 ± 7.9) [65]. It has been suggested that gait instability in SCA are characterized by a stronger effect of balance-related impairments of cerebellar control during slow walking and a stronger effect of impaired intra-limb coordination during fast walking [58]. Therefore, in clinical practice, it is necessary to evaluate not only the optimal gait speed, but also slow walking and fast walking, to extract the characteristics of gait instability.

3.3 Assessment of motor learning ability

The cerebellum has the ability to compensate for tissue damage and loss of function. This is called the cerebellar reserve [6]. Mitoma et al. suggested that this is important for motor rehabilitation at a time when the cerebellar reserve is functioning [6]. Motor rehabilitation in the early stages may maintain and improve the cerebellar reserve [66, 67]. Therefore, it is important to assess this parameter.

Cerebellar ataxia is the main symptom of SCA. Ataxia symptoms may represent a compensation for predictive control using feedback control [6]. Predictive control requires a mechanism called internal model [38]. The internal model is constantly updated by motor learning [68]. In turn, motor learning is one of the most important functions of the cerebellum. Thus, a measure of motor learning ability may be useful as an assessment of the cerebellar reserve.

Prism adaptation (PA) is widely used as an assessment of motor learning ability in patients with SCA [40, 69]. The basic procedure of PA is shown in **Figure 1**. First, at the "baseline," the task is performed without a prism lens. Subsequently, the prism lens is introduced and the task is performed. In the initial phase, the lens is set off to either the left or right side of the target, but the error is corrected as the number of repetitions increases. This period is called the "initial error correction phase." Thereafter, a spatial realignment phase is performed under the prism lens. The purpose of this phase is to gather visuospatial information including the errors. Next, the prism is removed and an "after-effect phase" is performed. If the spatial information is being re-learned, errors are generated in the opposite direction to the initial error correction phase. Recently, Hashimoto et al. developed the Adaptability Index (AI), which is a composite index computed from several parameters measured PA (**Figure 2**). The clinical efficacy of the AI in discriminating patients with SCA from healthy individuals has been demonstrated [70]. Furthermore, Bando et al. found that a reduced AI was correlated with gray matter atrophy in the cerebellum in the SCA group [49]. In particular, the right lobule VI and the left Crus I showed the most robust correlation. These cerebellar regions are consistent with the correlates of PA detected in previous human and nonhuman primate studies [71, 72]. AI is considered as a motor learning index that reflects the cerebellar reserve (in this case, the degree of cerebellar atrophy).

PA can be implemented using a simple system. In addition, it takes only 20 min to complete a PA. Reaching tasks can be performed even in the period during which

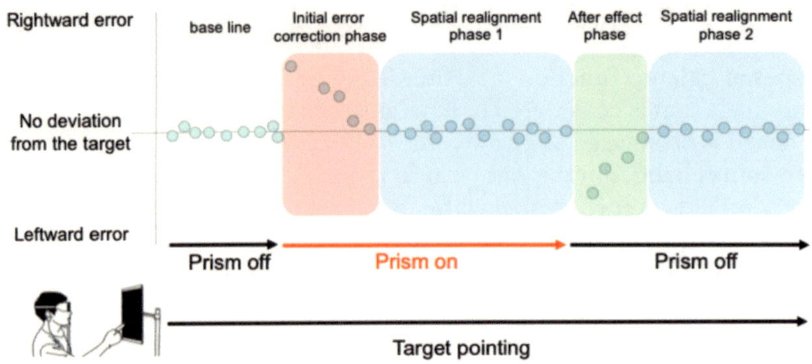

Figure 1.
Overview of prism adaptation. The ordinate shows the finger-touch error represented from the target to the touch point. Three phases are generally used: (1) absence of a prism lens (prism off), (2) presence of a prism lens (prism on), and (3) absence of a prism lens (prism off).

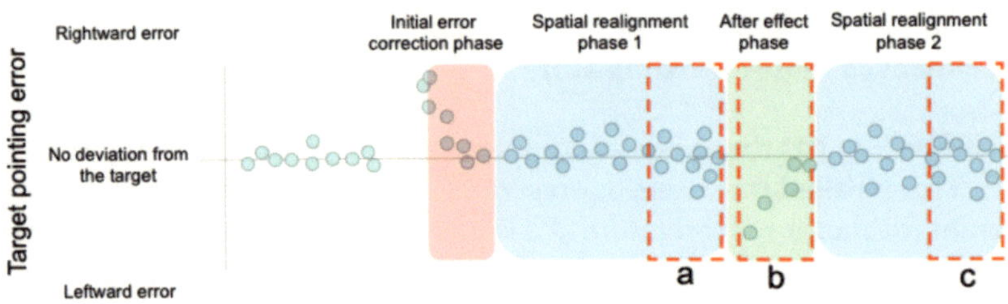

Figure 2.
Calculation of the adaptability index (AI). The AI is calculated as follows: AI = a × b × c, where "a" is the adaptation index defined as the probability of correct touches in the last 10 trials of the spatial realignment phase 1, "b" is the retention index defined as the probability of incorrect touches in the initial 5 trials of the after-effect phase, and "c" is the extinction index designated as the probability of correct touches in the last 10 trials of the spatial realignment phase 2.

the patient is unable to walk, and the fact that the PA can be assessed continuously over a long period is an advantage. However, only cross-sectional studies have been conducted in previous reports [40, 49, 69, 70, 73, 74]. Future studies need to be designed to examine long-term changes and intervention effects.

4. Rehabilitation

The targets of rehabilitation in cerebellar ataxia are mainly disability in ADL, gait, and motor dysfunction. Therefore, GAS, FIM, 10-m walking test, TCA, SARA, ICARS, and BESTest are used as important outcomes in rehabilitation. The most important strategies of rehabilitation for cerebellar ataxia including SCA consists in balance training (see Section 4.3), gait training (see Section 4.2), and muscle strengthening training using a high-intensity program (see Section 4.1). Further, optional possible interventions are using assistive technology (see Section 4.4) and neuromodulation technique (see Section 4.5).

4.1 Intensive and continuous training

Rehabilitation methods for cerebellar ataxia have been reported [75]. The most important strategy is the increase in the intensity of physical training, such as balancing, gait, and strength [76]. Several systematic reviews [77–79] and narrative reviews [3, 75, 80, 81] introduced and recommended intensive physical therapy for cerebellar ataxia in patients with SCA. Miyai et al. [62] reported that physical and occupational therapies of 2 h × 5 days +1 h × 2 days per week for 4 weeks were applied to inpatients and improved the SARA score and gait speed; however, the effect was carried over only up to 12 weeks after the training, and had disappeared at 24 weeks [62]. Conversely, Ilg et al. reported that intensive coordinative physiotherapy delivered over 4 weeks improved motor performance in degenerative cerebellar ataxia in a study with an intraindividual control design [63].

An outpatient rehabilitation program for 6 weeks applied to 19 participants with Friedreich's ataxia improved the motor domain item in the FIM score and Friedreich's Ataxia Impact Scale, but the posthome program could not maintain the effect [82]. Therefore, this finding indicates that continuous outpatient rehabilitation programs are important for maintaining the ADL in patients with Friedreich's ataxia. Additional large-scale studies are needed to investigate the long-term effect of outpatient rehabilitation programs and identify the characteristics of patients who respond to treatment. Therefore, the development of optimal individual programs is important to obtain the effect of training, regardless of the inpatient, outpatient, or home-self-training setting [83]. The semi-order program of the Research Committee for Ataxia Disease (Research team under the jurisdiction of the Ministry of Health, Labour and Welfare in Japan, http://ataxia.umin.ne.jp/rehabilitation/) can be used for this purpose.

Subsequently, the continuity of the intensive training is an important factor, because degradation in physical function was reported. Therefore, approaches aimed at upkeeping these programs in a way that suits the patients are needed. For example, exergames contribute to the practice of exercise at home. In the future, tele-rehabilitation systems [84] should be tested for the improvement (or maintenance) of the function and continuity of exercise.

4.2 Gait training

Gait training has been reported to improve spatiotemporal gait parameters (cadence, step length/width, gait speed, etc.) [85–87], complex gait (Timed Up and Go test, Dynamic Gait Index) [85], independence (FAC) [86], ataxia (SARA) [88], and adaptive locomotor adjustments (ALA) [88]. Patients with SCA exhibit problems other than the gait disturbance itself, i.e., stiffening of the body in an attempt to avoid the occurrence of gait disturbances. Therefore, it is important to focus on gait disturbances and increasing the number of walking patterns when considering gait training in a person with SCA.

Disturbances of gait are the core features of SCA [89–92], thus leading to a risk of falling down [93]. Patients with cerebellar ataxia walk with a reduced walking speed and cadence, as well as reduced step length, stride length, and swing phase; increased walking base width, stride time, step time, stance phase, and double limb support phase; and increased variability of step length, stride length, and stride time [94]. These items are affected by both balance-related impairments and deficits related to limb control and intra-limb coordination [95]. We believe that balance training and coordination training are key to the improvement of gait disturbances. Regarding the details of balance training, please refer to the Section 4.3.

In addition, stiffening of the body leads to a decrease in the number of walking patterns; as a result, ALA deteriorates [96, 97]. ALA implies that obstacle avoidance is achieved by modifying basic walking patterns in response to obstacle properties, e.g., a sloping road, stepping over an obstacle, or dynamically changing the spaces created by pedestrians in a hallway. In persons with SCA, feelings of anxiety as a result of the frequent experience of falls, as well as deficits related to limb control by ataxia, could negatively affect their ALA because of increased muscular co-contractions and reduced joint movements [98]. We will describe the approaches to improve ALA in the next paragraph.

The proposals for gait training are as follows: gait training without or with a treadmill. First, in gait training without a treadmill, we refer the reader to Section VI of the BESTest as gait adaptability training [61]. Section VI of the BESTest consists of a 7-item scale: (1) Gait Natural, (2) Change Speed, (3) Head Turns, (4) Pivot Turn, (5) Obstacles, (6) "Get Up & Go" Test, and (7) Cognitive Task "Get Up & Go" Test, aimed at evaluating the stability of the gait. These elements are important to improve ALA. As an example of gait training, persons with SCA are asked to walk while making an effort to change their walking speed according to therapist's instructions to engage is "fast (or slow)" walking as fast (or slow) as possible. If patients need assistance when walking, you might want to change the walking speed with the support of a therapist.

Second, gait training using a treadmill has advantages in that patients can practice a relatively large amount of gait training over a short period and the therapists can control the speed and incline easily. Gait training using a treadmill has been reported as a potentially promising tool for improving ALA in a person with SCA [88], as well as gait disturbances in a person with Parkinson's disease [99, 100]. It has been reported that variability was increased during slow and fast walking, but was normal during the preferred walking speed in a person with cerebellar ataxia [101]. Another study reported that, in ataxia, walking at the preferred speed minimizes the gait abnormalities, and the analysis of gait at a wide range of speeds is recommended [94]. For this reason, when using a treadmill in gait training, we suggest that walking be practiced at the speed at which the gait disturbance increases (i.e., slow or fast walking speed) for specific patients. When the fear of falling increases, the use of a harness is recommended, to provide a safe environment for gait without the fear of falling.

It is important to improve the balance ability and ALA during gait training in a person with SCA. Gait training is a relatively easy method; however, it is left to the therapist's discretion and experience. By changing the task itself or adjusting the difficulty level of the task, gait training may be able to overcome the limited walking patterns of these patients.

4.3 Balance training

All patients with SCA will develop balance difficulties during the course of the disease. Balance is essential for mobility, and is very important for QOL. Although there is no effective pharmacological treatment for decreasing the ataxia or slowing disease progression, physical therapy plays an important role in controlling ataxia and improving or maintaining function through training [76]. In general, the physical therapy programs for degenerative cerebellar ataxia are based on intensive static and dynamic balance and coordination training. There is some evidence that such therapeutic training programs alleviate the ataxic symptoms and improve functional activities in a person with cerebellar ataxia [63, 78, 102]. In these patients, the disease progressively damages the cerebellar structure that plays a crucial role in motor learning [103]; however, these studies have indicated that it is necessary for highly repetitive balance training for balance impairment in SCA. For this reason, highly repetitive balance training in patients with SCA should be the focus of future studies.

More concretely, balance training exercises in early stages of the disease, i.e., ambulation, include the following categories: (1) static balance training, (2) dynamic balance training, and (3) coordination training (**Figure 3**). In addition, combining a

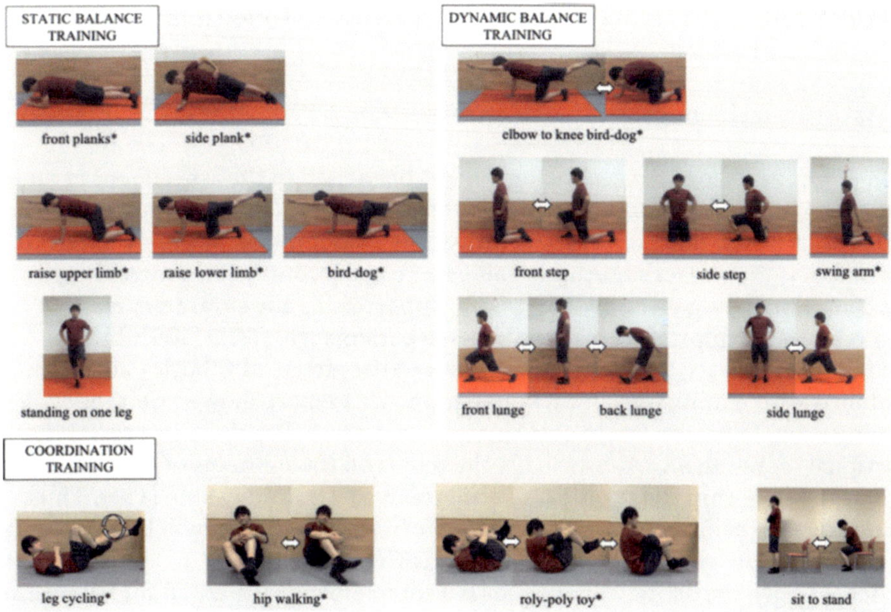

Figure 3.
National Center of Neurology and Psychiatry (NCNP) balance training program. This balance training program was devised through consultations with patients with SCA, medical doctors, and therapists at the NCNP in Japan. In the advanced stage of SCA, it is recommended to perform the programs indicated by an asterisk.

dual task with balance training improves balance and reduces the number of falls in individuals with cerebellar ataxia [104].

Moreover, it is important to provide support for these approaches and make them a habit of exercising. For instance, if the patients with SCA have no habit of exercising, they should start with a small number of exercises (i.e., the minimum necessary) to get used to exercising, followed by the gradual increase in the number of exercises. If the patients with SCA have a habit of exercising, the therapist should teach them to adjust the exercise load (e.g., exercise more slowly and/or provide a small base of support). It is also important to adopt balance training that can be enjoyed, e.g., video games [105] and Tai Chi [106], as a means of continuing balance training.

In advanced stages of the disease (i.e., no ambulation), it is necessary to perform balance training under safe conditions (e.g., prone, supine, crawl, and sitting positions), to prevent the decrease in physical activity. Even in advanced stages, it has been reported that a person with degenerative ataxia may benefit from balance training [107]. In addition, it is necessary to focus on ADL and living infrastructure at this stage. If a patient with SCA requires assistance during transfer, engaging in repetitive transfer training with assistance and/or modification of the living infrastructure (e.g., installation of handrails) are necessary.

Focusing on highly repetitive balance training in patients with SCA might preserve the balance function. There is no scientific basis for the number of balance training exercises that are necessary to achieve this goal; however, we would like to recommend engaging in 30 repetitions at least per balance training session. Furthermore, the balance training must be designed to provide a significant challenge to the person's balance. If a person with SCA wants to preserve the balance function, they have to continue engaging in repetitive balance training, "use it or lose it." However, few studies have reported the effect of gait and balance training in persons with SCA.

Therefore, further studies are needed to clarify the clinical effectiveness of gait and/or balance training.

4.4 Assistive technology

In recent years, various technologies have been used in the assessment of and treatment based on rehabilitation, as well as to support daily life in patients with SCD. Curara, a wearable robotic system, assists both hip and knee movements and supports the wearer's rhythmic gait using a synchronization control based on a central pattern generator [108]. Gait support using the curara system has been reported to improve gait smoothness in patients with SCD [109]. In addition to these findings, a recent study addressed the effects of robotic gait training combined with noninvasive brain stimulation. This report showed that robot gait training using Lokomat-Pro in combination with cerebellar tDCS improved the functional scores on SARA, especially the scores on the subitems of gait, stance, sitting, and heel-shin slide compared with robot gait training alone [110]. Thus, hybrid training using robots and noninvasive brain stimulation will be applied to the rehabilitation treatment of patients with SCD in the future.

Accordingly, the use of walking aids is a complementary method for balance and gait impairment. In general, walking aids such as canes and walkers improve postural stability, but their improper use increases the risk of falling [111]. Because the manipulation of a cane requires coordinated upper limb movements [112], patients with SCD who have upper limb ataxia are likely to experience difficulty in using a cane. Conversely, because a walker does not require much coordinated movement of the upper limbs, technology-based walkers are being developed. Recently, a smart walker for mobility assistance and monitoring system aid, ASBGo, was developed and reported to improve gait parameters and postural stability in patients with SCA [113, 114]. In addition to technology, some studies on walking assistance using dogs and handkerchiefs have also been reported. Walking with a rehabilitation dog that has been specifically trained for goal-directed interventions or with an assistance dog that helps people with physical disability and mobility impairments has been reported to improve balance while walking in patients with SCD [115]. Furthermore, the handkerchief-guided gait, in which the patient with SCD walks along with the caregiver while maintaining light tension on a handkerchief by pulling lightly, has been shown to decrease body swaying and increase stride length and gait velocity during walking [116].

Moreover, technology is also being used as a tool to assess ataxia in patients with SCD living at home. Most of them represent attempts to evaluate SARA, which is a typical measure of ataxia, at home. In recent years, a technology aimed at objectively evaluating the speech, upper and lower limb, balance, and gait functions using wearable inertial sensors and a Kinect camera was developed, which makes it possible to discriminate between normal and abnormal functions and to detect ataxia at an early stage [117]. In addition, SaraHome has been developed to allow the remote evaluation of SARA items using Kinect and Leap Motion Controller [118]. Moreover, a spoon equipped with an inertial sensor, called Ataxia Instrumented Measurement-Spoon, has been developed, which allows the evaluation of upper limb function in ataxia while eating with a spoon [119–121]. Because SCD is an intractable neurological disease, it is difficult for many patients to leave their houses. Therefore, the contribution of technology to home-based rehabilitation is expected to increase in the future if a low-cost and easy method of assessing ataxia at home is established using the technologies and products of daily living described above.

Regarding the support of ADL, BMI studies have been reported. Patients with severe SCA often have difficulty in communicating because of language impairment. The application of BMI using event-related potentials and frequency bands of EEG is being investigated as a solution to this problem. The operational accuracy of BMI using P300 for event-related potentials was 82.9% in patients with SCA, which was similar to the accuracy observed in healthy subjects (83.2%) [122]. There are also reports of BMI manipulation in patients with SCD using the EEG frequency band associated with motor imagery [123]. BMI has a wide range of applications in diseases of the central nervous system, such as communication tools, transportation, and life support, and is expected to contribute to the QOL of patients with SCD.

4.5 Neuromodulation

Neuromodulation via noninvasive brain stimulation (NIBS) is a potential method for the treatment of cerebellar ataxia [19, 124]. A previous systematic review [125] reported the effectiveness of cerebellar neuromodulation using the TMS technique of transcranial direct current stimulation (tDCS). The SARA and ICARS scores in patients with SCA3, multiple system atrophy, and postlesion ataxia, as assessed using real cerebellar rTMS (1 Hz), were significantly lower than those detected in the sham stimulation group [125]. Furthermore, no harmful side effects were noted [125]. Cerebellar rTMS can modulate the plasticity of the vestibular reflex [16, 126]; therefore, cerebellar rTMS has potential for application in balance training to enhance vestibular contributions.

A single session of anodal cerebellar tDCS (2 mA, 20 min) significantly improved SARA, ICARS, 9-hole-peg test, and 8-m walking test scores [127]. Furthermore, combined anodal cerebellar tDCS and cathodal spinal DCS (5 days/week, 2 weeks) improved SARA score, ICARS score, 9-peg test, and 8-m walking time in patients with degenerative cerebellar ataxia [128]. There is insufficient evidence regarding whether simultaneous stimulation is more effective than single stimulation [129]; however, it is possible that this intervention method will produce improvements. Based on these findings, which were gleaned from small-sample studies, we suggest that a neuromodulation montage will improve the ataxia, balance, and gait ability. Therefore, we should perform further studies using a larger population.

5. Conclusion

Individualized physical rehabilitation programs for patients with SCA may improve/maintain their motor function, balance, gait ability, and ADL. In particular, the intensity and continuity of gait and balance training need to be considered to achieve effectiveness. Furthermore, several technologies, such as depth sensors, robotics, and NIBS, have contributed to the development of methods for the assessment and treatment of motor dysfunction in individuals with SCA. We should continue to study populations suffering from dysfunction caused by SCA.

Acknowledgements

This work was supported by Shijonawate Gakuen University and JSPS KAKENHI (Grant Number 20 K11298).

Conflict of interest

The authors declare no conflict of interest.

Author details

Akiyoshi Matsugi[1*], Kyota Bando[2], Yutaka Kikuchi[3], Yuki Kondo[2] and Hideki Nakano[4]

1 Shijonawate Gakuen University, Daito, Osaka, Japan,

2 National Center of Neurology and Psychiatry, Kodaira, Tokyo, Japan

3 Institute of Brain and Blood Vessels Mihara Memorial Hospital, Isesaki, Gunma, Japan

4 Kyoto Tachibana University, Kyoto-city, Kyoto, Japan

*Address all correspondence to: a-matsugi@reha.shijonawate-gakuen.ac.jp

References

[1] Klockgether T, Mariotti C, Paulson HL. Spinocerebellar ataxia. Nat Rev Dis Primers. 2019;5(1):24. DOI:10.1038/s41572-019-0074-3

[2] Schmitz-Hubsch T, Coudert M, Giunti P, Globas C, Baliko L, Fancellu R, et al. Self-rated health status in spinocerebellar ataxia--results from a European multicenter study. Mov Disord. 2010;25(5):587-595. DOI:10.1002/mds.22740

[3] Pandolfo M, Manto M. Cerebellar and afferent ataxias. Continuum (Minneap Minn). 2013;19(5 Movement Disorders):1312-43. DOI:10.1212/01.CON.0000436158.39285.22

[4] Ilg W, Bastian AJ, Boesch S, Burciu RG, Celnik P, Claassen J, et al. Consensus paper: management of degenerative cerebellar disorders. Cerebellum. 2014;13(2):248-268. DOI:10.1007/s12311-013-0531-6

[5] Mitoma H, Manto M, Gandini J. Recent Advances in the Treatment of Cerebellar Disorders. Brain Sci. 2019;10(1). DOI:10.3390/brainsci10010011

[6] Mitoma H, Buffo A, Gelfo F, Guell X, Fuca E, Kakei S, et al. Consensus Paper. Cerebellar Reserve: From Cerebellar Physiology to Cerebellar Disorders. Cerebellum. 2020;19(1):131-153. DOI:10.1007/s12311-019-01091-9

[7] Mills RJ, Yap L, Young CA. Treatment for ataxia in multiple sclerosis. Cochrane Database Syst Rev. 2007(1):CD005029. DOI:10.1002/14651858.CD005029.pub2

[8] Trujillo-Martín MM, Serrano-Aguilar P, Monton-Alvarez F, Carrillo-Fumero R. Effectiveness and safety of treatments for degenerative ataxias: a systematic review. Mov Disord. 2009;24(8):1111-1124. DOI:10.1002/mds.22564

[9] Manto M, Gandini J, Feil K, Strupp M. Cerebellar ataxias: an update. Curr Opin Neurol. 2020;33(1):150-160. DOI:10.1097/WCO.0000000000000774

[10] Beaudin M, Matilla-Duenas A, Soong BW, Pedroso JL, Barsottini OG, Mitoma H, et al. The Classification of Autosomal Recessive Cerebellar Ataxias: a Consensus Statement from the Society for Research on the Cerebellum and Ataxias Task Force. Cerebellum. 2019;18(6):1098-1125. DOI:10.1007/s12311-019-01052-2

[11] Bodranghien F, Bastian A, Casali C, Hallett M, Louis ED, Manto M, et al. Consensus Paper: Revisiting the Symptoms and Signs of Cerebellar Syndrome. Cerebellum. 2016;15(3):369-391. DOI:10.1007/s12311-015-0687-3

[12] Ito M. Neurophysiological aspects of the cerebellar motor control system. Int J Neurol. 1970;7(2):162-176

[13] Manto M, Oulad Ben Taib N. The contributions of the cerebellum in sensorimotor control: what are the prevailing opinions which will guide forthcoming studies? Cerebellum. 2013;12(3):313-315. DOI:10.1007/s12311-013-0449-z

[14] Sharpe JA. Neurophysiology and neuroanatomy of smooth pursuit: lesion studies. Brain Cogn. 2008;68(3):241-254. DOI:10.1016/j.bandc.2008.08.015

[15] Tang SY, Shaikh AG. Past and Present of Eye Movement Abnormalities in Ataxia-Telangiectasia. Cerebellum. 2019;18(3):556-564. DOI:10.1007/s12311-018-0990-x

[16] Matsugi A, Yoshida N, Nishishita S, Okada Y, Mori N, Oku K, et al. Cerebellum-mediated trainability of eye and head movements for dynamic gazing. PLoS One.

2019;14(11):e0224458. DOI:10.1371/journal.pone.0224458

[17] Manto M, Bower JM, Conforto AB, Delgado-Garcia JM, da Guarda SN, Gerwig M, et al. Consensus paper: roles of the cerebellum in motor control--the diversity of ideas on cerebellar involvement in movement. Cerebellum. 2012;11(2):457-487. DOI:10.1007/s12311-011-0331-9

[18] Buckner RL. The cerebellum and cognitive function: 25 years of insight from anatomy and neuroimaging. Neuron. 2013;80(3):807-815. DOI:10.1016/j.neuron.2013.10.044

[19] Maas R, Helmich RCG, van de Warrenburg BPC. The role of the cerebellum in degenerative ataxias and essential tremor: Insights from noninvasive modulation of cerebellar activity. Mov Disord. 2020;35(2): 215-227. DOI:10.1002/mds.27919

[20] Ugawa Y, Uesaka Y, Terao Y, Hanajima R, Kanazawa I. Magnetic stimulation over the cerebellum in humans. Ann Neurol. 1995;37(6): 703-713. DOI:10.1002/ana.410370603

[21] Tanaka H, Matsugi A, Okada Y. The effects of imaginary voluntary muscle contraction and relaxation on cerebellar brain inhibition. Neurosci Res. 2017. DOI:10.1016/j.neures.2017.11.004

[22] Ilg W, Branscheidt M, Butala A, Celnik P, de Paola L, Horak FB, et al. Consensus Paper: Neurophysiological Assessments of Ataxias in Daily Practice. Cerebellum. 2018;17(5):628-653. DOI:10.1007/s12311-018-0937-2

[23] Matsugi A, Kikuchi Y, Kaneko K, Seko Y, Odagaki M. Cerebellar transcranial magnetic stimulation facilitates excitability of spinal reflex, but does not affect cerebellar inhibition and facilitation in spinocerebellar ataxia. Neuroreport. 2018;29(10):808-813. DOI:10.1097/WNR.0000000000001036

[24] Teo JT, Schneider SA, Cheeran BJ, Fernandez-del-Olmo M, Giunti P, Rothwell JC, et al. Prolonged cortical silent period but normal sensorimotor plasticity in spinocerebellar ataxia 6. Mov Disord. 2008;23(3):378-385. DOI:10.1002/mds.21847

[25] Restivo DA, Lanza S, Giuffrida S, Le Pira F, Drago MT, Di Mauro R, et al. Cortical silent period prolongation in spinocerebellar ataxia type 2 (SCA2). Funct Neurol. 2004;19(1):37-41

[26] Restivo DA, Lanza S, Saponara R, Rapisarda G, Giuffrida S, Palmeri A. Changes of cortical excitability of human motor cortex in spinocerebellar ataxia type 2. A study with paired transcranial magnetic stimulation. J Neurol Sci. 2002;198(1-2):87-92. DOI:10.1016/s0022-510x(02)00086-2

[27] Schwenkreis P, Tegenthoff M, Witscher K, Bornke C, Przuntek H, Malin JP, et al. Motor cortex activation by transcranial magnetic stimulation in ataxia patients depends on the genetic defect. Brain. 2002;125(Pt 2):301-309. DOI:10.1093/brain/awf023

[28] Oechsner M, Zangemeister WH. Prolonged postexcitatory inhibition after transcranial magnetic stimulation of the motor cortex in patients with cerebellar ataxia. J Neurol Sci. 1999;168(2):107-111. DOI:10.1016/s0022-510x(99)00164-1

[29] Nakashima K, Wang Y, Shimoda M, Sakuma K, Takahashi K. Prolonged silent periods produced by magnetic cortical stimulation in patients with cerebellar ataxia. Psychiatry Clin Neurosci. 1995;49(2):143-146. DOI:10.1111/j.1440-1819.1995.tb01879.x

[30] Matsugi A, Douchi S, Suzuki K, Oku K, Mori N, Tanaka H, et al. Cerebellar Transcranial Magnetic

Stimulation Reduces the Silent Period on Hand Muscle Electromyography During Force Control. Brain Sci. 2020;10(2). DOI:10.3390/brainsci10020063

[31] Nomura T, Takeshima T, Nakashima K. Reduced pre-movement facilitation of motor evoked potentials in spinocerebellar degeneration. J Neurol Sci. 2001;187(1-2):41-47. DOI:10.1016/s0022-510x(01)00522-6

[32] Matsugi A, Mori N, Uehara S, Kamata N, Oku K, Mukai K, et al. Task dependency of the long-latency facilitatory effect on the soleus H-reflex by cerebellar transcranial magnetic stimulation. Neuroreport. 2014;25(17):1375-1380. DOI:10.1097/WNR.0000000000000275

[33] Matsugi A, Mori N, Uehara S, Kamata N, Oku K, Okada Y, et al. Effect of cerebellar transcranial magnetic stimulation on soleus Ia presynaptic and reciprocal inhibition. Neuroreport. 2015;26(3):139-143. DOI:10.1097/WNR.0000000000000315

[34] Matsugi A, Okada Y. Cerebellar transcranial direct current stimulation modulates the effect of cerebellar transcranial magnetic stimulation on the excitability of spinal reflex. Neurosci Res. 2020;150:37-43. DOI:10.1016/j.neures.2019.01.012

[35] Kurokawa-Kuroda T, Ogata K, Suga R, Goto Y, Taniwaki T, Kira J, et al. Altered soleus responses to magnetic stimulation in pure cerebellar ataxia. Clin Neurophysiol. 2007;118(6):1198-1203. DOI:10.1016/j.clinph.2007.03.006

[36] Koster B, Deuschl G, Lauk M, Timmer J, Guschlbauer B, Lucking CH. Essential tremor and cerebellar dysfunction: abnormal ballistic movements. J Neurol Neurosurg Psychiatry. 2002;73(4):400-405. DOI:10.1136/jnnp.73.4.400

[37] Huang YZ, Chang YS, Hsu MJ, Wong AM, Chang YJ. Restoration of Central Programmed Movement Pattern by Temporal Electrical Stimulation-Assisted Training in Patients with Spinal Cerebellar Atrophy. Neural Plast. 2015;2015:462182. DOI:10.1155/2015/462182

[38] Honda T, Nagao S, Hashimoto Y, Ishikawa K, Yokota T, Mizusawa H, et al. Tandem internal models execute motor learning in the cerebellum. Proc Natl Acad Sci U S A. 2018;115(28):7428-7433. DOI:10.1073/pnas.1716489115

[39] Wong AL, Marvel CL, Taylor JA, Krakauer JW. Can patients with cerebellar disease switch learning mechanisms to reduce their adaptation deficits? Brain. 2019;142(3):662-673. DOI:10.1093/brain/awy334

[40] Hanajima R, Shadmehr R, Ohminami S, Tsutsumi R, Shirota Y, Shimizu T, et al. Modulation of error-sensitivity during a prism adaptation task in people with cerebellar degeneration. J Neurophysiol. 2015;114(4):2460-2471. DOI:10.1152/jn.00145.2015

[41] Schmitz-Hubsch T, Coudert M, Bauer P, Giunti P, Globas C, Baliko L, et al. Spinocerebellar ataxia types 1, 2, 3, and 6: disease severity and nonataxia symptoms. Neurology. 2008;71(13):982-989. DOI:10.1212/01.wnl.0000325057.33666.72

[42] Konczak J, Pierscianek D, Hirsiger S, Bultmann U, Schoch B, Gizewski ER, et al. Recovery of upper limb function after cerebellar stroke: lesion symptom mapping and arm kinematics. Stroke. 2010;41(10):2191-2200. DOI:10.1161/STROKEAHA.110.583641

[43] Bultmann U, Pierscianek D, Gizewski ER, Schoch B, Fritsche N, Timmann D, et al. Functional recovery and rehabilitation of postural impairment and gait ataxia in

patients with acute cerebellar stroke. Gait Posture. 2014;39(1):563-569. DOI:10.1016/j.gaitpost.2013.09.011

[44] Meira AT, Arruda WO, Ono SE, Neto AC, Raskin S, Camargo CHF, et al. Neuroradiological Findings in the Spinocerebellar Ataxias. Tremor Other Hyperkinet Mov (N Y). 2019;9. DOI:10.7916/tohm.v0.682

[45] Tada M, Nishizawa M, Onodera O. Redefining cerebellar ataxia in degenerative ataxias: lessons from recent research on cerebellar systems. J Neurol Neurosurg Psychiatry. 2015;86(8):922-928. DOI:10.1136/jnnp-2013-307225

[46] Ashburner J, Friston KJ. Voxel-based morphometry--the methods. Neuroimage. 2000;11(6 Pt 1):805-821. DOI:10.1006/nimg.2000.0582

[47] Burciu RG, Fritsche N, Granert O, Schmitz L, Sponemann N, Konczak J, et al. Brain changes associated with postural training in patients with cerebellar degeneration: a voxel-based morphometry study. J Neurosci. 2013;33(10):4594-4604. DOI:10.1523/JNEUROSCI.3381-12.2013

[48] Matsugi A, Kikuchi Y, Kaneko K, Seko Y, Odagaki M. Cerebellar transcranial magnetic stimulation facilitates excitability of spinal reflex, but does not affect cerebellar inhibition and facilitation in spinocerebellar ataxia. Neuroreport. 2018. DOI:10.1097/WNR.0000000000001036

[49] Bando K, Honda T, Ishikawa K, Takahashi Y, Mizusawa H, Hanakawa T. Impaired Adaptive Motor Learning Is Correlated With Cerebellar Hemispheric Gray Matter Atrophy in Spinocerebellar Ataxia Patients: A Voxel-Based Morphometry Study. Front Neurol. 2019;10:1183. DOI:10.3389/fneur.2019.01183

[50] Miterko LN, Baker KB, Beckinghausen J, Bradnam LV, Cheng MY, Cooperrider J, et al. Consensus Paper: Experimental Neurostimulation of the Cerebellum. Cerebellum. 2019;18(6):1064-1097. DOI:10.1007/s12311-019-01041-5

[51] Thach WT, Bastian AJ. Role of the cerebellum in the control and adaptation of gait in health and disease. Prog Brain Res. 2004;143:353-366. DOI:10.1016/s0079-6123(03)43034-3

[52] Miyai I. Challenge of neurorehabilitation for cerebellar degenerative diseases. Cerebellum. 2012;11(2):436-437. DOI:10.1007/s12311-011-0327-5

[53] Schmitz-Hubsch T, Tezenas du Montcel S, Baliko L, Boesch S, Bonato S, Fancellu R, et al. Reliability and validity of the International Cooperative Ataxia Rating Scale: a study in 156 spinocerebellar ataxia patients. Mov Disord. 2006;21(5):699-704. DOI:10.1002/mds.20781

[54] Schmitz-Hubsch T, Fimmers R, Rakowicz M, Rola R, Zdzienicka E, Fancellu R, et al. Responsiveness of different rating instruments in spinocerebellar ataxia patients. Neurology. 2010;74(8):678-684. DOI:10.1212/WNL.0b013e3181d1a6c9

[55] Schmahmann JD, Gardner R, MacMore J, Vangel MG. Development of a brief ataxia rating scale (BARS) based on a modified form of the ICARS. Mov Disord. 2009;24(12):1820-1828. DOI:10.1002/mds.22681

[56] Sullivan R, Yau WY, O'Connor E, Houlden H. Spinocerebellar ataxia: an update. J Neurol. 2019;266(2):533-544. DOI:10.1007/s00415-018-9076-4

[57] Honda T, Mitoma H, Yoshida H, Bando K, Terashi H, Taguchi T, et al. Assessment and Rating of Motor Cerebellar Ataxias With the Kinect v2 Depth Sensor: Extending Our Appraisal.

Front Neurol. 2020;11:179. DOI:10.3389/fneur.2020.00179

[58] Schniepp R, Schlick C, Pradhan C, Dieterich M, Brandt T, Jahn K, et al. The interrelationship between disease severity, dynamic stability, and falls in cerebellar ataxia. J Neurol. 2016;263(7):1409-1417. DOI:10.1007/s00415-016-8142-z

[59] Winser SJ, Smith C, Hale LA, Claydon LS, Whitney SL. Balance outcome measures in cerebellar ataxia: a Delphi survey. Disabil Rehabil. 2015;37(2):165-170. DOI:10.3109/09638288.2014.913709

[60] Kondo Y, Bando K, Ariake Y, Katsuta W, Todoroki K, Nishida D, et al. Test-retest reliability and minimal detectable change of the Balance Evaluation Systems Test and its two abbreviated versions in persons with mild to moderate spinocerebellar ataxia: A pilot study. NeuroRehabilitation. 2020. DOI:10.3233/NRE-203154

[61] Horak FB, Wrisley DM, Frank J. The Balance Evaluation Systems Test (BESTest) to differentiate balance deficits. Phys Ther. 2009;89(5):484-498. DOI:10.2522/ptj.20080071

[62] Miyai I, Ito M, Hattori N, Mihara M, Hatakenaka M, Yagura H, et al. Cerebellar ataxia rehabilitation trial in degenerative cerebellar diseases. Neurorehabil Neural Repair. 2012;26(5):515-522. DOI:10.1177/1545968311425918

[63] Ilg W, Synofzik M, Brotz D, Burkard S, Giese MA, Schols L. Intensive coordinative training improves motor performance in degenerative cerebellar disease. Neurology. 2009;73(22):1823-1830. DOI:10.1212/WNL.0b013e3181c33adf

[64] Ilg W, Seemann J, Giese M, Traschutz A, Schols L, Timmann D, et al. Real-life gait assessment in degenerative cerebellar ataxia: Toward ecologically valid biomarkers. Neurology. 2020;95(9):e1199-ee210. DOI:10.1212/WNL.0000000000010176

[65] Gouelle A, Megrot F, Presedo A, Husson I, Yelnik A, Pennecot GF. The gait variability index: a new way to quantify fluctuation magnitude of spatiotemporal parameters during gait. Gait Posture. 2013;38(3):461-465. DOI:10.1016/j.gaitpost.2013.01.013

[66] Fuca E, Guglielmotto M, Boda E, Rossi F, Leto K, Buffo A. Preventive motor training but not progenitor grafting ameliorates cerebellar ataxia and deregulated autophagy in tambaleante mice. Neurobiol Dis. 2017;102:49-59. DOI:10.1016/j.nbd.2017.02.005

[67] Fryer JD, Yu P, Kang H, Mandel-Brehm C, Carter AN, Crespo-Barreto J, et al. Exercise and genetic rescue of SCA1 via the transcriptional repressor Capicua. Science. 2011;334(6056):690-693. DOI:10.1126/science.1212673

[68] Kawato M, Ohmae S, Hoang H, Sanger T. 50 Years Since the Marr, Ito, and Albus Models of the Cerebellum. Neuroscience. 2020. DOI:10.1016/j.neuroscience.2020.06.019

[69] Fernandez-Ruiz J, Velasquez-Perez L, Diaz R, Drucker-Colin R, Perez-Gonzalez R, Canales N, et al. Prism adaptation in spinocerebellar ataxia type 2. Neuropsychologia. 2007;45(12):2692-2698. DOI:10.1016/j.neuropsychologia.2007.04.006

[70] Hashimoto Y, Honda T, Matsumura K, Nakao M, Soga K, Katano K, et al. Quantitative evaluation of human cerebellum-dependent motor learning through prism adaptation of hand-reaching movement. PLoS One. 2015;10(3):e0119376. DOI:10.1371/journal.pone.0119376

[71] Kuper M, Wunnemann MJ, ThurlingM,StefanescuRM,MaderwaldS, Elles HG, et al. Activation of the cerebellar cortex and the dentate nucleus in a prism adaptation fMRI study. Hum Brain Mapp. 2014;35(4):1574-1586. DOI:10.1002/hbm.22274

[72] Kitazawa S, Kimura T, Yin PB. Cerebellar complex spikes encode both destinations and errors in arm movements. Nature. 1998;392(6675):494-497. DOI:10.1038/33141

[73] Morton SM, Bastian AJ. Prism adaptation during walking generalizes to reaching and requires the cerebellum. J Neurophysiol. 2004;92(4):2497-2509. DOI:10.1152/jn.00129.2004

[74] Martin TA, Keating JG, Goodkin HP, Bastian AJ, Thach WT. Throwing while looking through prisms. II. Specificity and storage of multiple gaze-throw calibrations. Brain. 1996;119 (Pt 4):1199-1211. DOI:10.1093/brain/119.4.1199

[75] Matsugi A. Physical Therapy for Cerebellar Ataxia. In: Suzuki T, editor. Neurological Physical Therapy: IntechOpen; 2017. p. 158-173.

[76] Zesiewicz TA, Wilmot G, Kuo SH, Perlman S, Greenstein PE, Ying SH, et al. Comprehensive systematic review summary: Treatment of cerebellar motor dysfunction and ataxia: Report of the Guideline Development, Dissemination, and Implementation Subcommittee of the American Academy of Neurology. Neurology. 2018;90(10):464-471. DOI:10.1212/WNL.0000000000005055

[77] Fonteyn EM, Keus SH, Verstappen CC, Schöls L, de Groot IJ, van de Warrenburg BP. The effectiveness of allied health care in patients with ataxia: a systematic review. J Neurol. 2014;261(2):251-258. DOI:10.1007/s00415-013-6910-6

[78] Synofzik M, Ilg W. Motor training in degenerative spinocerebellar disease: ataxia-specific improvements by intensive physiotherapy and exergames. Biomed Res Int. 2014;2014:583507. DOI:10.1155/2014/583507

[79] Marquer A, Barbieri G, Pérennou D. The assessment and treatment of postural disorders in cerebellar ataxia: a systematic review. Ann Phys Rehabil Med. 2014;57(2):67-78. DOI:10.1016/j.rehab.2014.01.002

[80] Maring JR, Croarkin E. Presentation and progression of Friedreich ataxia and implications for physical therapist examination. Phys Ther. 2007;87(12):1687-1696. DOI:10.2522/ptj.20060232

[81] Lanza G, Casabona JA, Bellomo M, Cantone M, Fisicaro F, Bella R, et al. Update on intensive motor training in spinocerebellar ataxia: time to move a step forward? J Int Med Res. 2020;48(2):300060519854626. DOI:10.1177/0300060519854626

[82] Milne SC, Corben LA, Roberts M, Murphy A, Tai G, Georgiou-Karistianis N, et al. Can rehabilitation improve the health and well-being in Friedreich's ataxia: a randomized controlled trial? Clin Rehabil. 2018;32(5):630-643. DOI:10.1177/0269215517736903

[83] Keller JL, Bastian AJ. A home balance exercise program improves walking in people with cerebellar ataxia. Neurorehabil Neural Repair. 2014;28(8):770-778. DOI:10.1177/1545968314522350

[84] Dias JF, Oliveira VC, Borges PRT, Dutra F, Mancini MC, Kirkwood RN, et al. Effectiveness of exercises by telerehabilitation on pain, physical function and quality of life in people with physical disabilities: a systematic review of randomised controlled trials with GRADE recommendations.

Br J Sports Med. 2020. DOI:10.1136/bjsports-2019-101375

[85] Vaz DV, Schettino ReC, Rolla de Castro TR, Teixeira VR, Cavalcanti Furtado SR, de Mello Figueiredo E. Treadmill training for ataxic patients: a single-subject experimental design. Clin Rehabil. 2008;22(3):234-241. DOI:10.1177/0269215507081578

[86] Freund JE, Stetts DM. Use of trunk stabilization and locomotor training in an adult with cerebellar ataxia: a single system design. Physiother Theory Pract. 2010;26(7):447-458. DOI:10.3109/09593980903532234

[87] Im SJ, Kim YH, Kim KH, Han JW, Yoon SJ, Park JH. The effect of a task-specific locomotor training strategy on gait stability in patients with cerebellar disease: a feasibility study. Disabil Rehabil. 2017;39(10):1002-1008. DOI:10.1080/09638288.2016.1177124

[88] Fonteyn EM, Heeren A, Engels JJ, Boer JJ, van de Warrenburg BP, Weerdesteyn V. Gait adaptability training improves obstacle avoidance and dynamic stability in patients with cerebellar degeneration. Gait Posture. 2014;40(1):247-251. DOI:10.1016/j.gaitpost.2014.04.190

[89] Van de Warrenburg BP, Bakker M, Kremer BP, Bloem BR, Allum JH. Trunk sway in patients with spinocerebellar ataxia. Mov Disord. 2005;20(8):1006-1013. DOI:10.1002/mds.20486

[90] Globas C, du Montcel ST, Baliko L, Boesch S, Depondt C, DiDonato S, et al. Early symptoms in spinocerebellar ataxia type 1, 2, 3, and 6. Mov Disord. 2008;23(15):2232-2238. DOI:10.1002/mds.22288

[91] Rochester L, Galna B, Lord S, Mhiripiri D, Eglon G, Chinnery PF. Gait impairment precedes clinical symptoms in spinocerebellar ataxia type 6. Mov Disord. 2014;29(2):252-255. DOI:10.1002/mds.25706

[92] Choudhury S, Chatterjee S, Chatterjee K, Banerjee R, Humby J, Mondal B, et al. Clinical Characterization of Genetically Diagnosed Cases of Spinocerebellar Ataxia Type 12 from India. Mov Disord Clin Pract. 2018;5(1):39-46. DOI:10.1002/mdc3.12551

[93] Morton SM, Bastian AJ. Cerebellar control of balance and locomotion. Neuroscientist. 2004;10(3):247-259. DOI:10.1177/1073858404263517

[94] Buckley E, Mazzà C, McNeill A. A systematic review of the gait characteristics associated with Cerebellar Ataxia. Gait Posture. 2018;60:154-163. DOI:10.1016/j.gaitpost.2017.11.024

[95] Ilg W, Golla H, Thier P, Giese MA. Specific influences of cerebellar dysfunctions on gait. Brain. 2007;130(Pt 3):786-798. DOI.10.1093/brain/awl376

[96] Higuchi T. Visuomotor control of human adaptive locomotion: understanding the anticipatory nature. Front Psychol. 2013;4:277. DOI:10.3389/fpsyg.2013.00277

[97] McFadyen BJ, Fiset F, Charette C. Substituting anticipatory locomotor adjustments online is time constrained. Exp Brain Res. 2018;236(7):1985-1996. DOI:10.1007/s00221-018-5277-4

[98] Staab JP, Balaban CD, Furman JM. Threat assessment and locomotion: clinical applications of an integrated model of anxiety and postural control. Semin Neurol. 2013;33(3):297-306. DOI:10.1055/s-0033-1356462

[99] Pohl M, Rockstroh G, Rückriem S, Mrass G, Mehrholz J. Immediate effects of speed-dependent treadmill training on gait parameters in early Parkinson's

disease. Arch Phys Med Rehabil. 2003;84(12):1760-1766. DOI:10.1016/s0003-9993(03)00433-7

[100] Herman T, Giladi N, Hausdorff JM. Treadmill training for the treatment of gait disturbances in people with Parkinson's disease: a mini-review. J Neural Transm (Vienna). 2009;116(3):307-318. DOI:10.1007/s00702-008-0139-z

[101] Schniepp R, Wuehr M, Neuhaeusser M, Kamenova M, Dimitriadis K, Klopstock T, et al. Locomotion speed determines gait variability in cerebellar ataxia and vestibular failure. Mov Disord. 2012;27(1):125-131. DOI:10.1002/mds.23978

[102] Ilg W, Brötz D, Burkard S, Giese MA, Schöls L, Synofzik M. Long-term effects of coordinative training in degenerative cerebellar disease. Mov Disord. 2010;25(13):2239-2246. DOI:10.1002/mds.23222

[103] Paulson HL. The spinocerebellar ataxias. J Neuroophthalmol. 2009;29(3):227-237. DOI:10.1097/WNO0b013e3181b416de

[104] Winser S, Pang MYC, Rauszen JS, Chan AYY, Chen CH, Whitney SL. Does integrated cognitive and balance (dual-task) training improve balance and reduce falls risk in individuals with cerebellar ataxia? Med Hypotheses. 2019;126:149-153. DOI:10.1016/j.mehy.2019.03.001

[105] Ilg W, Schatton C, Schicks J, Giese MA, Schöls L, Synofzik M. Video game-based coordinative training improves ataxia in children with degenerative ataxia. Neurology. 2012;79(20):2056-2060. DOI:10.1212/WNL.0b013e3182749e67

[106] Winser SJ, Kannan P, Pang M, Smith C, Tsang WW. Potential Benefits and Safety of. J Altern Complement Med. 2018;24(12):1221-1223. DOI:10.1089/acm.2017.0396

[107] Schatton C, Synofzik M, Fleszar Z, Giese MA, Schöls L, Ilg W. Individualized exergame training improves postural control in advanced degenerative spinocerebellar ataxia: A rater-blinded, intra-individually controlled trial. Parkinsonism Relat Disord. 2017;39:80-84. DOI:10.1016/j.parkreldis.2017.03.016

[108] Tsukahara A, Yoshida K, Matsushima A, Ajima K, Kuroda C, Mizukami N, et al. Evaluation of walking smoothness using wearable robotic system curara(R) for spinocerebellar degeneration patients. IEEE Int Conf Rehabil Robot. 2017;2017:1494-1499. DOI:10.1109/ICORR.2017.8009459

[109] Tsukahara A, Yoshida K, Matsushima A, Ajima K, Kuroda C, Mizukami N, et al. Effects of gait support in patients with spinocerebellar degeneration by a wearable robot based on synchronization control. J Neuroeng Rehabil. 2018;15(1):84. DOI:10.1186/s12984-018-0425-4

[110] Portaro S, Russo M, Bramanti A, Leo A, Billeri L, Manuli A, et al. The role of robotic gait training and tDCS in Friedrich ataxia rehabilitation: A case report. Medicine (Baltimore). 2019;98(8):e14447. DOI:10.1097/MD.0000000000014447

[111] Bateni H, Maki BE. Assistive devices for balance and mobility: benefits, demands, and adverse consequences. Arch Phys Med Rehabil. 2005;86(1):134-145. DOI:10.1016/j.apmr.2004.04.023

[112] Lam R. Practice tips: choosing the correct walking aid for patients. Can Fam Physician. 2007;53(12):2115-2116

[113] Martins M, Santos C, Frizera A, Ceres R. Real time control of the ASBGo walker through a physical human–robot interface. Measurement. 2014;48:77-86. DOI:10.1016/j.measurement.2013.10.031

[114] Moreira R, Alves J, Matias A, Santos C. Smart and Assistive Walker - ASBGo: Rehabilitation Robotics: A Smart-Walker to Assist Ataxic Patients. Adv Exp Med Biol. 2019;1170:37-68. DOI:10.1007/978-3-030-24230-5_2

[115] Abbud G, Janelle C, Vocos M. The use of a trained dog as a gait aid for clients with ataxia: a case report. Physiother Can. 2014;66(1):33-35. DOI:10.3138/ptc.2013-17

[116] Nagumo K, Kunimi Y, Nomura S, Beppu M, Hirayama K. The handkerchief guide: a simple and practical method to improve ataxic gait in cerebellar subjects. Rinsho Shinkeigaku. 2015;55(5):311-319. DOI:10.5692/clinicalneurol.cn-000630

[117] Kashyap B, Phan D, Pathirana PN, Horne M, Power L, Szmulewicz D. Objective Assessment of Cerebellar Ataxia: A Comprehensive and Refined Approach. Scientific reports. 2020;10(1):9493. DOI:10.1038/s41598-020-65303-7

[118] Summa S, Schirinzi T, Bernava GM, Romano A, Favetta M, Valente EM, et al. Development of SaraHome: A novel, well-accepted, technology-based assessment tool for patients with ataxia. Comput Methods Programs Biomed. 2020;188:105257. DOI:10.1016/j.cmpb.2019.105257

[119] Nguyen KD, Corben LA, Pathirana PN, Horne MK, Delatycki MB, Szmulewicz DJ. An Instrumented Measurement Scheme for the Assessment of Upper Limb Function in Individuals with Friedreich Ataxia. Annu Int Conf IEEE Eng Med Biol Soc. 2019;2019:317-320. DOI:10.1109/EMBC.2019.8857107

[120] Nguyen KD, Corben LA, Pathirana PN, Horne MK, Delatycki MB, Szmulewicz DJ. The Assessment of Upper Limb Functionality in Friedreich Ataxia via Self-Feeding Activity. IEEE Trans Neural Syst Rehabil Eng. 2020;28(4):924-933. DOI:10.1109/TNSRE.2020.2977354

[121] Nguyen KD, Corben LA, Pathirana PN, Horne MK, Delatycki MB, Szmulewicz DJ. Assessment of Disease Progression in Friedreich Ataxia using an Instrumented Self Feeding Activity. Annu Int Conf IEEE Eng Med Biol Soc. 2020;2020:3827-3830. DOI:10.1109/EMBC44109.2020.9175980

[122] Okahara Y, Takano K, Komori T, Nagao M, Iwadate Y, Kansaku K. Operation of a P300-based brain-computer interface by patients with spinocerebellar ataxia. Clin Neurophysiol Pract. 2017;2:147-153. DOI:10.1016/j.cnp.2017.06.004

[123] Newman GI, Ying SH, Choi Y-S, Kim H-N, Presacco A, Kothare MV, et al., editors. Brain Computer Interface in Cerebellar Ataxia2010; Berlin, Heidelberg: Springer Berlin Heidelberg.

[124] Benussi A, Pascual-Leone A, Borroni B. Non-Invasive Cerebellar Stimulation in Neurodegenerative Ataxia: A Literature Review. Int J Mol Sci. 2020;21(6). DOI:10.3390/ijms21061948

[125] Franca C, de Andrade DC, Teixeira MJ, Galhardoni R, Silva V, Barbosa ER, et al. Effects of cerebellar neuromodulation in movement disorders: A systematic review. Brain Stimul. 2018;11(2):249-260. DOI:10.1016/j.brs.2017.11.015

[126] Matsugi A, Douchi S, Hasada R, Mori N, Okada Y, Yoshida N, et al. Cerebellar Repetitive Transcranial Magnetic Stimulation and Noisy Galvanic Vestibular Stimulation

Change Vestibulospinal Function. Front Neurosci. 2020;14:388. DOI:10.3389/fnins.2020.00388

[127] Benussi A, Koch G, Cotelli M, Padovani A, Borroni B. Cerebellar transcranial direct current stimulation in patients with ataxia: A double-blind, randomized, sham-controlled study. Mov Disord. 2015;30(12):1701-1705. DOI:10.1002/mds.26356

[128] Benussi A, Dell'Era V, Cantoni V, Bonetta E, Grasso R, Manenti R, et al. Cerebello-spinal tDCS in ataxia: A randomized, double-blind, sham-controlled, crossover trial. Neurology. 2018;91(12):e1090-ee101. DOI:10.1212/WNL.0000000000006210

[129] Matsugi A. Reader response: Cerebello-spinal tDCS in ataxia: A randomized, double-blind, sham-controlled, crossover trial. Neurology. 2019;92(23):1121. DOI:10.1212/WNL.0000000000007623

Chapter 6

Living and Coping with Spinocerebellar Ataxia: Palliative Care Approach

Caroline Bozzetto Ambrosi and Patricia Bozzetto Ambrosi

Abstract

The discussion about the palliative care approach in spinocerebellar ataxia (SCA) has become extremely relevant. Mainly after considering that most progressive ataxias are incurable, there are few published studies on their palliative and end-of-life care. Although many patients with degenerative neurological diseases have a normal life expectancy, some forms of SCA (e.g., type 1, 2, 3, and 17) can progress rapidly, with a shorter life span. This chapter will discuss current guidelines and recommendations that have been drawn from the broader field of progressive neurological conditions. In addition, we also review aspects of strategic end-of-life care management, the involvement of the multidisciplinary team and the contribution of allied health professionals are essential for excellent patient support care in a palliative approach. More studies on your supportive care and end-of-life care to manage this serious illness to improve quality of life and reduce suffering, addressing complex medical symptoms, psychosocial issues, general well-being, and planning strategies for better living and coping are needed.

Keywords: spinocerebellar ataxia, palliative care, supportive care, end-of-life, wellness being, medical strategies

1. Introduction

> *"We cannot avoid suffering but we can choose how to cope with it, find meaning in it, and move forward with renewed purpose."* (Viktor E Frank)

> *"Our most cruel failure in how we treat the sick and the elderly is the failure to recognize that they have priorities beyond just being safe and living longer; that the chance to shape one's history is essential to sustaining the meaning of life; that we can reshape our institutions, our culture and our conversations in ways that transform the possibilities of the last chapters of everyone's life."* (Atul Gawande)

Spinocerebellar ataxia (SCA) is a term that refers to a group of inherited autosomal dominant ataxias characterized by degenerative changes in the part of the brain related to movement control (cerebellum) and in the spinal cord, its connections with progressive decline in functional capacity [1–3].

The significant improvement in the classification and correlation of the clinical profile of the different forms of cerebellar ataxias is due to genetic advances in medical diagnosis. Although several subtypes of SCAs have been identified, phenotypically, cerebellar ataxia is a common feature of each type with individual differences regarding mutations in many different genes and the involvement of the cerebellum and its connections [3–10].

On the other hand, despite these advances in genetics, modifying therapies targeting specific genes or stem cells, there is no current definitive treatment able to stop the progression of most cases as in most degenerative neurological diseases. Strategic management of SCA to improve quality of life and reduce suffering, addressing complex medical symptoms, psychosocial issues, general well-being, and planning requires a broad and dedicated multidisciplinary involving palliative care approach. For patients with more complex needs help from a palliative care specialist team may be necessary [11–24].

In this chapter, it would be reviewed the main clinical aspects, the perspectives of therapeutic management, directed symptomatic management, support, and multidisciplinary team including the current guidelines regarding patients living and coping with SCA.

2. Recognition and key clinical aspects

Genetically and phenotypically, several subtypes of SCAs have been identified. Cerebellar ataxia is a feature of each type; other distinguishing features may suggest a specific type. However, more than ⅔ of patients with SCA have mutations at known loci that can be identified through genetic testing. In addition, among patients with apparently idiopathic sporadic cerebellar ataxia (no family history), an SCA mutation (types 1, 2, 3, 6, 7, 8, or 12; most often SCA-6) or Friedreich's ataxia can be identified in approximately ¼ of patients [1–4, 10, 25].

In most subtypes of SCAs (SCA 1, 2, 3, 6, 7, and 17) a genetic abnormality will be identified related to the expansion of CAG repeats in the region that encodes the polyglutamine tracts in protein products, like what is observed in Huntington's disease. Wild-type chromosomes with a stable CAG repeat have 6–34 repeat units; more than 36 repeats result in an unstable, expanded, disease-causing allele.

Clinically disorders associated with CAG repeat expansion share several relevant medical condition features [6, 7]:

1. Middle age beginning with progressive ataxia, neuronal dysfunction, and eventual neuronal loss over the next 10–20 years.

2. The greater the number of CAG repeats in expanded alleles, the earlier the age of onset and the more severe the disease.

3. Repeats show somatic and germinal instability. Then, successive generations of affected families experience the anticipation, a phenomenon characterized by earlier onset and a progressively worse phenotype in subsequent generations.

4. Only a certain subset of neurons is vulnerable to dysfunction, although the relevant protein is widely expressed throughout the brain and other tissues.

5. Cerebellar atrophy is the most reported finding. Brainstem atrophy is variable, being more characteristic of SCA types 1, 2, and 7.

6. Neurodegeneration of the tegmental pontine reticular nucleus has been reported in patients with SCA types 1, 2, and 3; this nucleus plays a role in the performance of smooth horizontal searching eye movements and the accuracy of the horizontal saccade.

3. Perspectives of medical palliative care management

The nihilistic view of the treatment of SCA, as it happens for long past years with many other neurodegenerative diseases, is no longer justified. In addition to rehabilitation therapies, there are specific complications to be looked for and treated. These interventions can significantly alleviate the problems of progressive ataxia and prevent potentially fatal complications. An enthusiastic, motivational, and well-informed medical approach in addition to follow-up by a multidisciplinary team can provide valuable support to a patient with SCA. When a patient approaches the end-of-life, specialized palliative care services should be involved to help to meet their specific needs as will be described in this chapter [20–24, 26–33].

4. Symptomatic management

A patient living with SCA, the care team services should be involved to help to meet their specific symptomatic needs. A variety of potential symptoms will need to be managed as treatment "strategies" are often derived from other neurological conditions with similar symptoms and work equally well.

The approach to treating spasticity and bladder symptoms, for example, is the same as for people with other neurological diseases [22, 23]. The assessment and management of these complications is best done by involving therapy specialists, and the work of the multidisciplinary team can improve patient care. Speech and language therapy are essential along the patient's journey, from monitoring the swallowing function in the initial stages and providing useful tips on how to avoid complications, to planning feeding by percutaneous gastrostomy [24].

The impact of cerebellar disease on cognition is not widely known, but it can have a significant impact on morbidity. These "remote" effects of cerebellar dysfunction can include frontal subcortical impairments affecting personality, behavior, and judgment.

Mental health complications (anxiety, depression) can exacerbate people's sense of isolation nowadays with Covid-19 pandemic and fear of the future. These symptoms often accompany sleep disturbances and fatigue but are barely recognized [26].

Management of cardiac complications is especially important in Friedreich's ataxia; it can be applied to SCA and patients need regular electrocardiographic checks and echocardiograms to detect the development of cardiomyopathy. Echocardiography may show concentric left ventricular hypertrophy (possibly in more than half of cases, especially early-onset ones).

As the disease progresses, hypertrophy regresses, resulting in a thin, dilated left ventricle. Cardiac enzymes may be asymptomatically elevated (in the absence of arrhythmia or acute coronary syndrome) and may help to have baseline values for future comparison. It is essential to involve an experienced cardiologist with knowledge in the treatment of neuromuscular disorders, initially to advise on medications to treat cardiomyopathy and heart failure, and later to manage arrhythmias and other complications related [27, 28].

5. Multidisciplinary team work

The multidisciplinary team is clearly important in evaluating and managing patients with SCA. Patients with SCA should be offered several times a year's reviews, ideally by a specialized team including a neurologist, advanced palliative care, nurse, and when it would be necessary, other members as social workers, psychiatrists, therapists, physiatrists.

Speech and linguistic therapy (for both communication and feeding), occupational therapy, and physiotherapy can each make important contributions at different stages of the patient's life. Patients require regular review to identify any new symptoms that may need treatment, and for patients to take advantage of advances in diagnosis and any newly available treatments [20–24].

These multidisciplinary interventions can significantly alleviate the problems of progressive ataxia and prevent potentially fatal complications. An enthusiastic and well-informed medical approach in addition to follow-up by a multidisciplinary team can provide valuable support to an SCA's patient.

In addition, those with no established cause for their ataxia can undergo a thorough and repeated review of the clinical features and investigation results, which sometimes leads to a clearer diagnosis. Patients and their families should be encouraged to contact patient support groups. When a family first receives the diagnosis of progressive ataxia, patients are usually not heard of the condition or come across other people with it. Support from patient organizations can, therefore, be particularly important at this stage. The possibility of meeting others in the same situation, receiving emotional support and information, and the opportunity to learn about research developments can all help [30, 33].

6. Supportive care

Given that most cases of SCA are difficult to manage, can progress rapidly and have a shortened life. Studies on their palliation and end-of-life care are needed. Most of the recommendations in guidelines at present are drawn from the broader field of other progressive neurological conditions. The supportive care comes alongside your current medical and neurology team to give an extra layer of support not only for patients but also for family [29–32].

Palliative care is for anyone living with a serious illness at any stage and can be offered at any facility wherever the patient is at the hospital, clinic outpatients, and at home [30]. To provide support to physical and psychological symptoms, social issues, community groups, talking about end-of-life worries, other issues (for example, copying distress) and spiritual concerns. Compared to usual care, it provides relief from suffering, works in quality of life, plans for decline, advances care planning, focuses on patient and family, and requires a consistent team approach and strategy. The members of neuro-palliative care are doctors who are going to review the history and physical examination, establishing goals of care, symptoms management and education, about disease and prognosis discussion which is very difficult related to SCA due to lack of key markers then normally is done about the point of care of each individual case.

The nursing team is going to make the medication review, identification of medical durable power of attorney, discussion of advanced care planning at the appropriate time besides for screening caregiver distress. The chaplain is going to address spiritual/existential concerns, exploring social and family issues, identifying, and discussing grief and screening for caregiver distress. The social worker is going to advice on financial and insurance issues. Providing resources for home health care, and logistical aspects of transition care.

7. Planning care and final remarks

As stated in our book and described in several chapters, the symptoms of ACS are much more than ataxia or movement disorders and include variability in cognitive complaints, mood disorders, fatigue, vision problems, problems eating, swallowing, neuropathy, cramps, muscle, heart, intestinal, and urinary problems among many others.

The psychiatrist Viktor Frankl identified three main sources for meaning in care and life [31]:

- At work, doing something significant.

- In love, caring for another person. *The salvation of man is through love and in love*.

  In a position of utter desolation, when a man cannot express himself in positive action, when his only achievement may consist in enduring his sufferings in the right way—an honorable way—in such a position man can, through loving contemplation of the image he carries of his beloved, achieve fulfillment.

  Love goes very far beyond the physical person of the beloved. It finds its deepest meaning in his spiritual being, his inner self.

- In courage during difficult times. Suffering itself is meaningless, but our response to it gives it meaning.

Then understating an individual's value goals of care allows clinical to align the care with what is the most important to the patients with SCA and their families. Mainly addressing the value goals of care, for example, doing exploration about what was life before SCA? and other several important matters, asking questions about the quality of life and hoping to realize what is most important for the patient. Patients with intractable and/or distressing physical symptoms may benefit from referral for a specialist palliative care, which might also help those with complex social, psychological, or spiritual needs and plan of care.

The time for planning end-of-life care is when the clinician answers 'No' to the 'surprise question'—'Would you be surprised if this patient died in the next 12 months?'—as well there being generic and specific (for ataxia) indicators that the patients have reached the terminal phase of their illness. Management in this phase should be geared toward enabling a 'good death': being treated as an individual, with dignity and respect, without pain or other distressing symptoms, in familiar surroundings, and the company of close friends and family.

The plan of care will be a negotiation of goals of care and realistic medical options for management. Besides that, the unique psychosocial stressors such as changing roles in a relationship, loss of autonomy, financial strain, communication difficulties, social isolation (especially during Covid-19 pandemic), cosmetic effects, a social stigma that will require referral to an attorney, psychotherapy, support groups, ataxia specific programming in rehabilitation centers.

The spiritual distress includes grief, guilt, fear of cognitive decline, existential crisis, and death anxiety and needs to be addressed the caregiver distress as well as high levels of burden and depression. Establishing an advance care plan to ensure that patient wishes are known and planning the future associated with improvement of patient satisfaction, lower hospital admission rates, decreases significantly the psychological comorbidities and suffering for the family.

Having a diagnosis of SCA is very important to identify a care team to strategize how to bring back meaning to life, getting extra support at home, and community resources Also, despite care holistic symptom management, long-term relationship with the care team, and establishing a plan for future advanced care planning [30, 32, 33].

In conclusion, the palliative care approach in patients living and coping with SCA should benefit the patient's life in many aspects, such as better quality of life, improved symptom burden, better life of patient and family, greater satisfaction with care, higher rates and quality of the advance plan of future and no adverse effects. In addition to that, further studies are needed as clinical priorities included to develop and implement models to integrate palliative care into neurology and to develop and implement informative quality measures to evaluate and compare palliative approaches in SCA through validated trials.

Conflict of interest

The authors declare no conflict of interest or disclosures.

Author details

Caroline Bozzetto Ambrosi[1] and Patricia Bozzetto Ambrosi[2*]

1 Medical Doctor, Specialist in Palliative Care, United Kingdom

2 Medical Doctor, Alumni Sorbonne University, France

*Address all correspondence to: patriciabozzettoadm@outlook.com

References

[1] Harding AE. Clinical features and classification of inherited ataxias. Advances in Neurology. 1993;**61**:1

[2] Whaley NR, Fujioka S, Wszolek ZK. Autosomal dominant cerebellar ataxia type I: A review of the phenotypic and genotypic characteristics. Orphanet Journal of Rare Diseases. 2011;**6**:33

[3] Cloak MU. The wide spectrum of spinocerebellar ataxias. Cerebellum. 2005;**4**:2

[4] Schols L, Szymanski S, Peters S, et al. Genetic background of apparently idiopathic sporadic cerebellar ataxia. Human Genetics. 2000;**107**:132

[5] Trottier Y, Lutz Y, Stevanin G, et al. Polyglutamine expansion as a pathological epitope in Huntington's disease and four dominant cerebellar ataxias. Nature. 1995;**378**:403

[6] Jacobi H, Bauer P, Giunti P, et al. The natural history of spinocerebellar ataxia types 1, 2, 3, and 6: A 2-year follow-up study. Neurology. 2011;**77**:1035

[7] Rüb U, Bürk K, Schöls L, et al. Damage to the reticular tegmental nucleus of the pons in spinocerebellar ataxia type 1, 2, and 3. Neurology. 2004;**63**:1258

[8] Diallo A, Jacobi H, Cook A, et al. Survival in patients with spinocerebellar ataxia types 1, 2, 3, and 6 (EUROSCA): A longitudinal cohort study. Lancet Neurology. 2018;**17**:327

[9] Jacobi H, du Montcel ST, Romanzetti S, et al. Conversion of individuals at risk for spinocerebellar ataxia types 1, 2, 3, and 6 to manifest ataxia (RISCA): The longitudinal cohort study. Lancet Neurology. 2020;**19**:738

[10] Orr HT, Zoghbi HY. Trinucleotide repeat disorders. Annual Review of Neuroscience. 2007;**30**:575

[11] Sullivan R, Yau WY, O'Connor E, Houlden H. Spinocerebellar ataxia: An update. Journal of Neurology. 2019;**266**:533

[12] Tang B, Liu C, Shen L, et al. Frequency of SCA1, SCA2, SCA3/MJD, SCA6, SCA7, and DRPLA CAG trinucleotide repeat expansion in patients with hereditary spinocerebellar ataxia from Chinese kindreds. Archives of Neurology. 2000;**57**:540

[13] Geschwind DH, Perlman S, Figueroa CP, et al. The prevalence and wide clinical spectrum of spinocerebellar ataxia type 2 trinucleotide repeat in patients with autosomal dominant cerebellar ataxia. American Journal of Human Genetics. 1997;**60**:842

[14] Moseley ML, Benzow KA, Schut LJ, et al. Incidence of dominant spinocerebellar and Friedreich triplet repeats among 361 ataxia families. Neurology. 1998;**51**:1666

[15] Orr HT, Chung MY, Banfi S, et al. Expansion of an unstable trinucleotide CAG repeat in spinocerebellar ataxia type 1. Nature Genetics. 1993;**4**:221

[16] Skinner PJ, Koshy BT, Cummings CJ, et al. Ataxin-1 with an expanded glutamine tract alters nuclear matrix-associated structures. Nature. 1997;**389**:971

[17] Klement IA, Skinner PJ, Kaytor MD, et al. Ataxin-1 nuclear localization and aggregation: Role in polyglutamine-induced disease in SCA1 transgenic mice. Cell. 1998;**95**:41

[18] Zoghbi HY, Orr HT. Pathogenic mechanisms of a polyglutamine-mediated neurodegenerative disease, spinocerebellar ataxia type 1. The Journal of Biological Chemistry. 2009;**284**:7425

[19] Chiara C, Giannini C, Adinolfi S, et al. The AXH module: An independently folded domain common to ataxin-1 and HBP1. FEBS Letters. 2003;**551**:107

[20] Gehrking KM, Andresen JM, Duvick L, et al. Partial loss of Tip60 slows mid-stage neurodegeneration in a spinocerebellar ataxia type 1 (SCA1) mouse model. Human Molecular Genetics. 2011;**20**:2204

[21] Lam YC, Bowman AB, Jafar-Nejad P, et al. ATAXIN-1 interacts with the Capicua repressor in its native complex to cause SCA1 neuropathology. Cell. 2006;**127**:1335

[22] Khan F, Amatya B, Bensmail D, et al. Non-pharmacological interventions for spasticity in adults: An overview of systematic reviews. Annals of Physical and Rehabilitation Medicine. 2019;**62**(4):265-273. DOI: 10.1016/j.rehab.2017.10.001

[23] Fowler CJ, Panicker JN, Drake M, et al. A UK consensus on the management of the bladder in multiple sclerosis. Journal of Neurology, Neurosurgery, and Psychiatry. 2009;**80**:470-477. DOI: 10.1136/jnnp.2008.159178

[24] Logemann JA. Evaluation and Treatment of Swallowing Disorders. American Journal of Speech-Language Pathology. Vol. 6. College Hill Press; 1998. pp. 395-400. DOI: 10.1097/00020840-199812000-00008

[25] Storey E, du Sart D, Shaw JH, et al. Frequency of spinocerebellar ataxia types 1, 2, 3, 6, and 7 in Australian patients with spinocerebellar ataxia. American Journal of Medical Genetics. 2000;**95**:351

[26] Hoche F, Guell X, Vangel MG, et al. The cerebellar cognitive affective/Schmahmann syndrome scale. Brain. 2018;**141**:24870. DOI: 10.1093/brain/awx317

[27] Weidemann F, Liu D, Hu K, et al. The cardiomyopathy in Friedreich's ataxia—New biomarker for staging cardiac involvement. International Journal of Cardiology. 2015;**194**:50-57. DOI: 10.1016/j.ijcard.2015.05.074

[28] Writing Committee Members, Yancy CW, Jessup M, et al. 2013 ACCF/AHA guideline for the management of heart failure: A report of the American College of cardiology Foundation/American Heart Association Task Force on practice guidelines. Circulation. 2013;**128**:e240-e327. DOI: 10.1161/CIR.0b013e31829e8776

[29] Ellershaw J, Ward C. Care of the dying patient: The last hours or days of life. BMJ. 2003;**326**:30-34

[30] Byrne J et al. Palliative Care in Neurological Disease: A Team Approach. 1st edition. CRC Press; 2009

[31] Frankl VE. Palliative Care in Neurology. Ebook in English

[32] Voltz R et al. Palliative Care in Neurology. Contemporary Neurology Series. Illustrated edition. Oxford University Press; 12 August 2004

[33] Creutzfeldt CJ, Kluger B, Kelly AG, Lemmon M, Hwang DY, Galifianakis NB, et al. Neuropalliative care: Priorities to move the field forward. Neurology. 2018;**91**(5):217-226. DOI: 10.1212/WNL.0000000000005916